Springer Series on Nursing Management and Leadership

Joyce J. Fitzpatrick, PhD, RN, FAAN, Series Editor

Advisory Board: Pamela Cipriano, PhD, RN, FAAN; Harriet R. Feldman, PhD, RN, FAAN; Greer Glazer, RN, PhD, CNP, FAAN; Daniel J. Pesut, PhD, APRN, BC, FAAN; Elaine La Monica Rigolosi, EdD, JD, FAAN

D1366975

About the Author

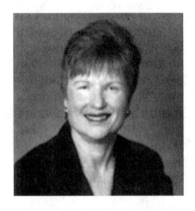

The author knows about nursing challenges because she has experienced them. June Fabre has worked as a clinical nurse, educator, and manager in many specialties such as medical surgical, psychiatry, home care, long-term care, ambulatory care, managed care, rehabilitation, and cardiology. She decided to turn the challenges of working as a nurse into an opportunity—to start a business focused on producing positive health care change. Ms. Fabre believes that nurses can create positive change by supplementing their comprehensive medical knowledge with communication and leadership techniques.

Ms. Fabre is an author, speaker, and consultant on various topics such as critical thinking, high-performance teams, and the art of creating a staff-friendly culture. As a result, she has spoken to audiences, large and small, all across the country. In addition, she has published more than 30 articles in popular health care journals. Ms. Fabre received her RN and BS in education from State University College, Plattsburgh, NY; a BSN from Excelsior College, Albany, NY; and an MBA from Plymouth State College, Plymouth, NH. For more information, you can reach Ms. Fabre at *www.junefabre.com.*

JUNE FABRE, MBA, RNC

SMART
NURSING

HOW TO CREATE A POSITIVE WORK ENVIRONMENT THAT EMPOWERS AND RETAINS NURSES

SPRINGER PUBLISHING COMPANY

NURSING MANAGEMENT & LEADERSHIP SERIES

Springer Publishing Company, Inc.
11 West 42nd Street
New York, NY 10036

Acquisitions Editor: Ruth Chasek
Production Editor: J. Hurkin-Torres
Cover design by Mimi Flow

06 07 08 09 / 5 4 3

Library of Congress Cataloging-in-Publication Data

Fabre, June.
  Smart nursing : how to create a positive work environment that empowers and retains nurses / by June Fabre.
    p. ; cm. — (Springer series on nursing management and leadership)
    ISBN 0-8261-2585-9
    1. Nursing services—United States—Personnel management. 2. Nursing services—United States—Administration. 3. Nurses—Supply and demand—United States. 4. Nurses—United States—Social conditions. 5. Manpower planning—United States.
      [DNLM: 1. Nursing—methods. 2. Nursing—organization & administration. 3. Medical Errors—prevention & control. 4. Nurse's Role. 5. Nurse-Patient Relations. 6. Patient Satisfaction.] I. Title. II. Series.
    RT89.3.F33 2005
    610.73'068'3—dc22   2004031097

Printed in the United States of America by Bang Printing.

The anecdotal cases in this book are composites of nursing experiences from US and international nurses combined with hypothetical situations. The names used in the cases have been disguised.

To my parents

Fritz Bendel and Olga Bendel, LPN (Retired),
who lived and loved the American Dream

Contents

Contributors

Jeannette Ives Erickson, RN, MS, is senior vice president for patient care and chief nurse at Massachusetts General Hospital, Boston, MA.

Linda Pullins, RN, is vice president for patient care at Marion General Hospital in Marion, OH.

Nancy M. Valentine, RN, PhD, D.Sc. (Hon.), MSN, MPH, FAAN, FNAP, is national nursing executive at CIGNA HealthCare, Medical Strategy and Health Policy, in Hartford, CT.

Acknowledgments

Writing a book is a process that requires the assistance of others, and I would like to recognize the people who have helped me along the way.

A special thank-you to all of the members of the Derry Writers Group, especially Janet Buell, J. Richard Reed, Roger Davies, and Dennis Hett. J. Richard Reed introduced me to the Derry Writers Group where I learned to write for publication. I'd also like to express my appreciation to the Author's Guild, NYC, and the New Hampshire Writers Project for the support and education that they provide to authors.

Various nurses read portions of my manuscript, suggested examples to use, or assisted me in determining the best way to present important nursing issues. These wonderful nurses are Suzanne Belanger, Anne Smith, Gerri Gowlis, Marilyn Asselin, Byrdie Jo Baker, Laura Rapp, Deborah O'Neil, Kathryn Deneault, Louise McGourty, Sigrid Kuriger, Yvette Moquin, Elaine St. Pierre, and my sister, Joan Livingston. Their education and experience include LPN, RN, RNC, ARNP, MSN, MBA, and PhD. Their broad perspectives help me with my goal—that *Smart Nursing* provide information needed by all nurses.

And I appreciate those who generously contributed to *Smart Nursing*:

- Jeanette Ives Erickson, RN, MS, chief nurse, Massachusetts General Hospital, Boston, Massachusetts.
- Nancy M. Valentine, RN, Ph.D., D.Sc.(Hon.), MSN, MPH, FAAN, FNAP, national nursing executive, CIGNA HealthCare, Medical Strategy and Health Policy, Hartford, Connecticut.
- Linda Pullins, RN, vice president for patient care, Marion General Hospital, Inc., Marion, Ohio.

- Librarians Ruslyn Vear, Head of Research at the Amherst Town Library and Dorothy Y. Kameoka from the Dorothy M. Breen Memorial Library who helped a great deal with my research. And I appreciate the editorial suggestions that I received from Prill McGann, Janice Borzendowski, and my editor at Springer, Ruth Chasek.
- My family, my husband Grant, my daughters Michelle, Kim, and Sherri, and Andrew White for their patience, flexibility, and sense of humor. I also appreciate the warm support and guidance of Rev. Susan A. Henderson and the members of the Womens Spirituality Group at the Amherst Congregational Church.
- Colleagues at the organizations where I am a member: The National Speakers Association especially Dianna Booher, MA, CSP, CPAE, Booher Consultants, Inc., Grapevine, Texas, and W. Mitchell, CSP, CPAE, Mitchell Communications, Santa Barbara, California.
- Every single member of the National Speakers Association–New England for their continuous caring, warm support, and friendship for so many years.
- The American Organization of Nurse Executives and the Massachusetts Organization of Nurse Executives, the American Nurses Association and the New Hampshire Nurses Association. Your friendship and leadership role modeling has been appreciated very much.

Part I

Why Use Smart Nursing?

Introduction

In "Jack and the Beanstalk," the mythical beanstalk grows and allows Jack to enter a mysterious world of peril and adventure, the land of the giant and his extraordinary riches. Within this land is a goose that lays golden eggs.

Health care managers face a similar situation. They also live with peril and adventure, especially while staffing their facilities. They have golden geese, but don't always recognize them. Their golden geese come disguised as nurses. Organizations are figuratively killing their nurses with negative working conditions and actively ignoring their contributions. Nurses are one of health care's greatest assets, health care gold.

In the 1990s, health care management slashed staff instead of performing the precise surgery needed to decrease waste. Nurses could not survive in this new environment of overuse so they either burned out or found other careers. Now health care facilities face sinking financial futures because of the nursing shortage. Nursing costs have increased, and some facilities have been forced to put expansion plans on hold. Bottom lines have declined and facilities have not been able to offer necessary services to their communities.

Negative cultures also interfere with nurses' needs. A lack of courtesy and respect chips away at a nurse's sense of self, destroying his or her energy and motivation. Some organizations have also endangered nurses' physical needs by being slow to adopt safer equipment such as needleless IV systems because it is expensive. They have violated Maslow's second basic need: safety and security.

Caring people, not policies and procedures, determine whether patients receive quality health care services. Many of these caring people are nurses. Unfortunately, the nursing shortage threatens

3

worldwide health care systems. An article in *The Wall Street Journal* cited a study from the *New England Journal of Medicine* (Needleman, Beurhaus, Mattke, Stewart, and Zeleuinsky, 2002) in highlighting the seriousness of this shortage: "When there are too few registered nurses at bedsides, patients are significantly more likely to suffer serious complications, such as urinary-tract infections, internal bleeding, and even death" (as cited in Johannes, 2002). Moreover, nurses are being overworked yet underutilized, ignored, and even censured for speaking up; the result is that patient safety is being compromised. An editorial in *The New York Times*, referring to a report in the *Journal of the American Medical Association* (Aiken, Clarke, Silbur, and Sloane, 2002), addressed this aspect of the problem:

> When hospital nurses are given too many patients to care for, the patients have a much greater risk of dying. Adding a single patient to a nurse's caseload seems to increase the risk of dying within 30 days by 7 percent.

The solution is not to ask, or expect, nurses to work faster; rather, we must enable them to work *smarter*, by removing obstacles that interfere with their productivity. *Smart Nursing* was written with the express purpose of explaining how to do that. It encourages clinical nurses and managers to work together using conceptual, communication, and leadership approaches.

Smart Nursing is more than the title of this book; it is also a system of strategies that enables nurses to use their *full professional capacity* to deliver safe patient care in a variety of clinical settings. At the same time, it empowers managers to work with staff more effectively. Indeed, the wisdom behind these strategies is that they blend health care knowledge with business expertise. More than helping nurses to maximize the "nursing process" with commitment, competence, and compassion, the Smart Nursing strategies also address the bottom line for managers. In short, the dollar difference between the present level of nurse productivity and a nurse's full professional capacity is the potential cost savings that Smart Nursing offers. Organizations often justify their treatment of nurses by suggesting that financial constraints are forcing their actions, but research and experiential data show the opposite. The Advisory Board in Washington, D.C., estimates that a 500-bed hospital can save $800,000 a year by cutting its nurse turnover by a mere 3% (Nursing Executive Center, 2000).

CONCEPTUAL FRAMEWORK OF SMART NURSING

Smart Nursing and the nursing process are based on general systems theory, which researchers discovered years ago to be the most effective way to study human processes in fields such as psychology, sociology, and political science. General systems theory seeks to understand the "wholeness" of any system by understanding the interdependence of its parts.

Smart Nursing strategies promote the wholeness of the health care system. It assists organizations to synergize components of good management practices using six basic elements: respect, simplicity, flexibility, integrity, communication, and professional culture. These components form the basis of Smart Nursing and can only exist when organizations are willing to use long-term strategies to preserve them.

Too many health care organizations are using short-term fixes—Band-Aid solutions—that exacerbate the nursing shortage. It is long-term strategies, Smart Nursing strategies, such as building relationships and effective communication that deliver better results.

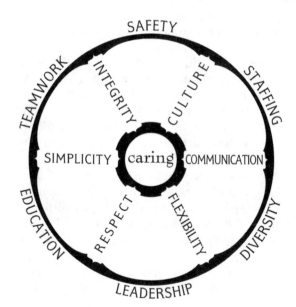

FIGURE 1   The Smart Nursing model.

Smart Nursing is based on these assumptions:

- Nurses are an essential part of a health care facility's investment.
- Systems problems are preventing nurses from performing at their full professional capacity.
- Restoring nursing value by considering nurses as assets and treating them as valued professionals maximizes the return on an organization's human resource investment.
- Organizations that provide environments where nurses can perform at their best attract and retain the best people.
- Leaders and managers are more effective when they build strong relationships with their staff.
- Long-term strategies such as effective communication and staff-friendly cultures enable organizations to achieve the best results.
- Combining sound clinical practices with ethical business actions produces the safest and most cost-effective patient care.
- Positive relationships among health care professionals generate energy and raise productivity.
- Clinical nurses who can make decisions at the patient level save management time and increase patient satisfaction.
- Individuals who embrace lifelong learning develop the ability to thrive in a rapidly changing world.

Everyone—consumers, business executives, the government, and nurses themselves—is alarmed at the high rate of medical errors and the failing health care system. Now is the right time for change. Now is the right time for nurses and managers to learn to work together. And now is the right time for health care organizations to take better care of one of their most important resources—their nurses.

Smart Nursing describes practical techniques that every nurse, manager, and organization can use to restore patient safety, reduce nurse turnover, and stimulate realistic health-care solutions. Throughout, solid data from business and health care sources are used, yet the book is written in an easy-to-understand style, to ensure its accessibility to readers, whether they are chief nurses, managers, RNs, LPNs; nonnurse professionals such as physicians, CEOs, or trustees; or consumers interested in learning how to improve health care.

Chapter 1

Relationships:
The Importance of a
Staff-Friendly Culture

The key to unleashing the organization's potential to excel is putting that power in the hands of the people who perform the work.

—James M. Kouzes

You, the nurse manager, arrive at your office at 8:00 on Monday morning. Stephanie, one of your most competent nurses, asks for a few minutes of your time. She hands you a letter of resignation. She is the third RN to do so in the last 60 days.

Even as you consider ways to fill the holes in the schedule, you wonder why she is leaving. After all, the nurses have just received a substantial pay raise and they have the best benefit package in the area. Managers and nonnurses remark that the nurses are getting everything they want but never seem to be satisfied.

As for yourself, you must address what is becoming a vicious cycle of nurse resignations and overtime for the remaining staff, which you know will lead to more nurse burnout and more resignations.

But from Stephanie's point of view, the reasons she resigned are all too apparent. Consider how one of her workdays develops:

1. She arrives for work and discovers that she will be short-staffed.
2. During the course of the day, she encounters disrespectful behavior and asks herself why she bothers. The source of this disrespectful behavior is usually physicians or managers. Occasionally it comes from other nurses or staff. Patients are usually respectful and the prime source of much of the support that nurses receive.
3. She has no time for a break because of the heavy workload, causing her to be exhausted early and less effective as the day wears on.
4. During a staff meeting, she makes some suggestions that would improve care, but management tables them, leaving her frustrated and angry.
5. There are several patient admissions that afternoon, but the staff has the attitude of every nurse for herself, each struggling to finish her work and unwilling to lend a hand where it's needed.

At the end of the day, certain tasks that would have made a big difference to patients remain undone, and Stephanie leaves work feeling that the patients received poor care. In sum, it was another in a long series of *energy-draining* days that add up to Stephanie's decision to finally throw in the towel.

It doesn't have to be like this. In a staff-friendly culture, nurses have a completely different experience—an *energy-enhancing* experience. Though their workload is substantial, they find they can do it effectively and efficiently. They are treated as important professionals. They can say, and mean, "We don't do rude here." Their suggestions at the last staff meeting have been given full consideration and will be implemented the same week. They feel they are part of a high-performance team, one that can handle multiple admissions easily by working cooperatively. They feel good physically, as well, because despite the heavy activity on the unit, they are encouraged to make time for meals and breaks. Thus, they leave work tired but satisfied, safe in the knowledge that their hard work had meaning and resulted in excellent patient care.

Nurses are your organization's best revenue sources. Nurses *generate revenue* by delivering excellent patient care. When patients choose a health care facility, they want safety and a personal connection with staff members; nurses satisfy both of these needs.

Nurses generate revenue when their personal connections keep patients coming back to your facility. These connections do not necessarily take a lot of time. It is not the time that's important; it is the quality of the connections and the skill with which they are made.

For example: While preparing to perform an admission assessment, a nurse notices that the patient is having an important conversation with a family member. She shows compassion by telling the patient she will return in 15 minutes for the assessment. Time spent: 30 seconds. The result is invaluable patient appreciation and satisfaction. This provides a source for future revenue flow.

Staffing issues are more easily resolved in a staff-friendly culture because there is a spirit of collaboration, humor, and cooperation.

For example: A nurse wants to avoid working a weekend double shift. As she and several peers wait for the weekly staff meeting to begin, she asks one of them to substitute for her, commenting, "I will be so sad if you can't do it." She uses the opportunity for some humorous persuasion as well. She turns to another peer and says, "Do you want to see how sad we will be if you don't work on Saturday? See our sad faces!" The staff has a good belly laugh, and the nurse successfully covers the shift. And the shift is covered at straight time, not premium pay, so it turns out to be a money-saving solution as well.

Staff-friendly cultures are very cost effective because staff can spend 100% of their time and energy doing their work instead of wasting time and energy surviving a dysfunctional system. If a nurse earns $50,000 but has to waste 25% of her time dealing with unnecessary conflict and petty political agendas, you lose $12,500 of the nursing value for each nurse. With only 16 nurses, that adds up to a lost value of $200,000 a year. And the negative culture decreases nurse satisfaction and increases staff turnover. The cost of staff turnover can add hundreds of thousands of dollars to that $200,000. Can we afford to continue wasting nurse resources this way?

A LONG-TERM PERSPECTIVE

Long-term strategies prevail in staff-friendly cultures. Long-term strategies of respect, relationships, and collaboration provide an environment where staff can thrive. These long-term strategies can transform our current health care environment from chaos into an environment of consistent quality and safety.

According to a 2003 honesty and ethics Gallup poll, people respect nurses more highly than any other profession, surpassing physicians, teachers, and dentists (Gallup, 2003). Health care organizations should show respect for nurses by giving them the power to control their practice, the credit from management for their accomplishments, and the opportunities to utilize their skills fully.

Improved relationships create productive employees who are committed to their organizations. Management and nurses build relationships when they give praise for work well done and consistently practice honesty and trust. This enables them to collaborate and work as partners. Health care is a relationship business. It is built on relationships between caregivers and patients, as well as on relationships between caregivers and health care providers. However, nursing productivity is often measured only in the number of tasks a nurse can accomplish. That's like going to the store and buying apples and then trying to judge your success by counting how many oranges you have.

Many facilities rely heavily on sign-on bonuses and optimistic recruitment ads. These techniques attract nurses to the facility, but those same nurses usually leave when their commitment expires. Or they resign when they realize the facility wasn't all it had been described to be. These are short-term fixes.

Consider the folly of too many quick fixes. Suppose a 2-year-old has a tantrum. Occasionally giving in to the child's demands probably won't cause any harm. However, using the quick fix and always giving in to those demands will produce a monster. Health care has created its own monster by using the quick fix much too often. This Band-Aid approach has left a reservoir of unresolved issues: frustrated and burned-out employees, dissatisfied patients, and wasted resources.

Staff recruitment and retention improve with Smart Nursing strategies. Patients enjoy high-quality care, and nurses can maintain patient safety. Patient quality and safety improve because nurses who report safety concerns are valued and considered to be credible reporters. Then, nurses are assured that when they report their safety concerns, action will be taken in time to prevent medical errors and deaths. Reducing complications and unnecessary deaths, of course, benefits patients and their families. But it also benefits health care facilities because their reputation improves. With more patients, revenue increases, improving the bottom line. Nurses are renewable resources with substantial value, but not when management burns them out.

Ann O'Sullivan, MSN, RN, testifying before the Senate Governmental Affairs committee on behalf of the American Nurses' Association had this to say:

> Nurses are, understandably, reluctant to accept positions in which they will face inappropriate staffing, be confronted by mandatory overtime, inappropriately rushed through patient care activities and face retaliation if they report unsafe practices. (O'Sullivan, 2001)

Nurses are powerless. Even during nursing shortages, facilities waste nurses. They waste nursing time, ignore nursing potential, and destroy nursing spirit. Many organizations value tasks but ignore nurses' ideas and opinions.

For example, a nurse observes symptoms of physical decline in a patient—the patient's respiratory rate is 40 when a normal respiratory rate for an adult is 20. Her assessment rules out hyperventilation and anxiety, which if present would indicate less significant reasons for rapid respirations. This nurse is very concerned that the patient is having early symptoms of a major medical problem and reports her observations to the charge nurse, supervisor, and physician. She asks for additional diagnostic tests to be done. Her request is refused, and no one takes action because the patient's other vital signs are normal. An hour later the patient's respiratory rate continues to be rapid and the nurse reports her concerns a second time. She again asks for additional tests. But those who have the power to take action ignore the nurse's concerns because they don't value her professional judgment. Nurses only have the power to continue assessing and reporting, not to order additional diagnostic tests or medication. Eventually, the patient goes into cardiac arrest and the rest of the team finally jumps into action. Additional testing is finally done during the resuscitation process, but it is done too late and the patient dies. This is an example of a "failure to rescue" event, as described in recent research (Nurse Staffing Levels and the Quality of Care in Hospitals, Needleman, Buerhaus, Mattke, Stewart, & Zeleuinsky, 2002). The nurse recognized the symptoms early, but those who had the power to act did not take those early symptoms of complications seriously.

In the midst of the nursing shortage, nurses often don't even have the extra time for frequent patient assessments when they are concerned about a patient. For example, a patient's medical order may require vital sign assessment every 4 hours. But if a nurse is concerned about a patient's condition, he may want to recheck the patient's vital signs every 30 minutes for a short while. However, with his heavy assignment, there is no time to follow through on more frequent vital signs. His other responsibilities (treatments and medications) consume all of his time, so he may miss the early symptoms of major complications.

Patients appreciate nurses' compassion because it contributes so much quality to their health care services, but others disregard it. Nursing management has little influence in the power game, and this leaves nurses with no voice at all.

Clinical nurses and managers need to teach others how to treat them with respect. There are various ways to accomplish this, and your choices depend on your own personal style.

- Be assertive about ending disrespectful behavior. If someone is rude, bring it to his or her attention assertively, and make it clear that disrespectful behavior will not be tolerated.
- Insist that supervisors and physicians take timely action when you notice a patient in physical decline. It is unacceptable for patients to suffer with unnecessary medical decline.
- Document everything you do and say accurately, completely, and professionally.
- Take appropriate pride in the skillful assessments and astute observations that prevent patients from having unnecessary physical decline. Patients usually acknowledge your value, but managers and physicians frequently do not. This is not conceit. It is taking pride in a job well done.

In their book *From Silence to Voice*, Bernice Buresh and Suzanne Gordon (2000) say that nurses should not just sit at the tables of power. They should be listened to and respected for their views. Quality care demands nurses' influence and voice.

For example, nurses may need more staff or updated equipment, but may be preempted by the budgetary requests of those with more power. Because money is scarce, nursing input is often *not* viewed as a priority and is therefore the last to be taken into consideration.

Management and physicians often hear reports of valid problems and treat them as complaints. Whistle-blowers are treated harshly. In their 2001 study of nurses, Harvard researchers (Tucker, Edmonson, & Spear) observed the difficulty that nurses encountered when they tried to report significant information:

> We did not observe any instances where the nurse contacted someone about a trivial or insignificant exception. In fact, we observed several occasions where we were surprised that the nurse did *not* raise awareness around a problem that we felt could have serious consequences. (p. 135)

When nurses are concerned about a patient's physical decline, they are often disregarded, even if they express their concern through the proper channels. Nurses can't call physicians who work in the emergency room because it is against protocol. The protocol represents a valid and safe system in most cases. Physicians, as independent practitioners or as part of a group practice, do not usually examine each other's patients unless there is a conversation between them first. Many times when this conversation happens, an order is written arranging for examination of the patient and the patient receives the necessary care.

When the conversation doesn't happen, nurses can be left with a deteriorating patient and no way to intervene. In such cases, the patient would receive better care anyplace *except* in a hospital. Consider how one patient was denied proper care in the following example.

In one instance, several concerned nurses tried to facilitate a physician-to-physician conversation so that the emergency room physician could examine an inpatient who was in physical decline. During one of these situations, a very frustrated nurse suggested humorously to a colleague, "Why don't we get the patient dressed, put him in a wheelchair, and then wheel him into the emergency room's front door with the following comment: 'We found this guy lying outside in the parking lot. He looks sick. Can you check him over?'" Such humor releases stress when nurses are powerless.

This problem has been partially addressed by using hospitalists, physicians whose job responsibilities include examining hospitalized patients. However, not all hospitals use hospitalists, and not all physicians ask them to care for their patients.

Other situations reveal the way that vital nursing observation builds partnerships with physicians. For instance, a nurse looked at a physician order for insulin. It seemed different than usual. She expressed her concern to a peer and a supervisor, but they weren't concerned. Still, her intuition, based on many years of experience, urged her to call the physician. After she read the order, the physician said, "Thank you for *thinking*. This order is wrong." The physician corrected the order, and a potential medication error was averted. It's that easy. Simple respectful conversations are one of the ways to prevent serious medical errors. Why don't we use this method more often?

HEALTH CARE PROBLEMS ARE OPPORTUNITIES

Health care problems are one side of the coin. Problems are also opportunities—opportunities for staff nurses, managers, and physicians to engage in Smart Nursing practices.

Smart Nursing amplifies nurse effectiveness by providing training in critical thinking, assertiveness, leadership, and communication. Public speaking and writing for publication are also an important part of the mix. With Smart Nursing, nurses learn to describe their full professional value quantitatively as well as qualitatively.

Workloads for health care professionals will not decline. If anything, they will increase. But Smart Nursing strategies enable nurses to manage heavy workloads without burn-out. The whole medical team will then be working in synergy. Synergy occurs when the total team effort exceeds the sum of each person's efforts working individually.

A positive environment is the foundation of high productivity because it allows nurses to access their higher selves. You probably have had experience using your higher self during particularly harmonious periods of your life. Think back to when you were working on a project you especially enjoyed. Recall your energy level. You wanted to spend more time on your project, didn't you? And the time you spent working seemed more like play than work. You were accessing your higher self and capable of achieving more work than usual. It's the same for nurses working in a staff-friendly culture. Contrast this to when you were involved in unsatisfactory work. Time dragged, and you felt like procrastinating and putting the work off as long as possible. That's how the present atmosphere saps nurse productivity.

Gary Zukav puts it this way in his book, *The Seat of the Soul*: "When we align our thoughts, emotions and actions with the highest part of ourselves, we are filled with enthusiasm, purpose and meaning. Life is rich and full. . . . We are joyously and intimately engaged with our world" (Zukav, 1989, p. 26).

Are you are a manager, clinical nurse, or a person interested in learning how the nursing crisis affects patient care? You can help turn the nursing crisis into an opportunity. You can improve the treatment of nurses. And you can improve medical care for yourself, your loved ones, and your community.

A NURSE LEADER IN ACTION

Jeannette Ives Erickson, RN, MS
Senior vice president for patient care and chief nurse
Massachusetts General Hospital

Building Bridges: A Strategy for Success

As the chief nurse of the Massachusetts General Hospital, I am surrounded by the best and brightest clinical nurses and leadership in nursing. I believe the reason for our success is that we always remember why we became nurses. Our commitment to nursing has guided us in creating an agenda for MGH nursing that is aligned with our own personal values and passion for the profession.

Three Cornerstones for Success

When I assumed the role of chief nurse just over 5 years ago, I immediately worked with my leadership team to create the three cornerstones for MGH nursing: a shared vision, guiding principles, and long-term strategic goals.

  1. ***Shared vision:*** *We hold a shared picture of the future we seek to create.*

---

2. ***Value statements or guiding principles:*** *We believe in the worth of what we have and through our desire to create something new. Our value statements influence strategic planning because they are the result of staff decisions and behaviors. The true test of our values occurs when our staff—and more important, our patients—can see and feel those values in action.*

3. ***Long-term strategic goals:*** *Long-term objectives are the measure of departmental and organizational effectiveness. They are not quick fixes. They are high-leverage, long-term strategies that create fundamental change and solutions.*

Create Bridges Between Management and Nursing

These three cornerstones paved the way for strategic planning. I have seen many strategic plans end up in colorful binders with great graphics, but covered with dust from lack of use. They do not come alive. I was committed to making certain that MGH nursing's strategic plan came alive.

I see strategic planning as an opportunity to create a bridge between clinical nurses and management. Both management and clinical nurses are necessary to fulfill our vision. Clinical nurses have both formal and informal opportunities to provide input into the strategic plan and to assess how it's going.

Examples of How We Create Bridges

1. *I meet with a staff nurse representative from every clinical unit each month at our Staff Nurse Advisory Committee. This committee forms a bridge between clinical nurses and management so that we can work together as partners to solve health care dilemmas.*

2. *We use an annual survey called the Staff Perception Survey of Professional Practice Environment. It is sent to clinical nurses throughout MGH, which queries them about their feelings of autonomy, control over practice, collaborative relationships, and perceptions about what's working and not working.*

3. *Through ongoing staff forums and clinical rounds, staff voice their perceptions about their practice.*
4. *We obtain leadership input through formal meetings and quarterly retreats where we critically review where we are going and how we are going to get there.*

Prepare Staff for Strategic Planning

Our strategic plan resonates with clinical nurses and leadership because their voices are heard and incorporated into it. We make an investment of time and energy to prepare staff to be able to participate actively in strategic planning. However, the dividends are high. Every member of the Department of Nursing feels ownership of our strategic direction. And clinical nurses and leadership see evidence that they are being heard because the strategic plan is written in their words. Together, we translate the plan into action.

These are the vision statement, guiding principles, and long-term strategic goals we generated at MGH:

Vision Statement

As nurses, health professionals, and patient-care-services support staff, our every action is guided by knowledge, enabled by skill, and motivated by compassion. Patients are our primary focus, and the way we deliver care reflects that focus every day. We believe in creating a practice environment that has no barriers, is built on a spirit of inquiry, and reflects a culturally competent workforce that is supportive of the patient-focused values of this institution. It is through our professional practice model that we make our vision a demonstrable truth every day by letting our thoughts, decisions, and actions be guided by our values. As clinicians, we ensure that our practice is caring, innovative, scientific, and empowering, and is based on a foundation of leadership and entrepreneurial teamwork.

Guiding Principles

We are ever alert for opportunities to improve patient care; we provide care based on the latest **research findings**.

*We recognize the importance of **encouraging** patients and families to participate in the decision affecting their care.*

*We are most effective as a team; we continually strengthen our relationship with each other and actively promote **diversity** within our staff.*

*We enhance patient care and the systems supporting that care as we work with others; we eagerly enter new **partnerships** with people inside and outside the Massachusetts General Hospital.*

*We never lose sight of the needs and expectations of our patients and their families as we make clinical decisions based on the most **effective** use of internal and external resources.*

*We view **learning** as a lifelong process essential to the growth and development of clinicians striving to deliver quality patient care.*

*We acknowledge that maintaining the **highest standards** of patient-care delivery is a never-ending process that involves the patient, family, nurses, all health care providers, and the community at large.*

Long-Term Strategic Goals

Enhance communication to promote employees' understanding of organizational imperatives and their involvement in clinical decisions that affect their practice.

Promote and advance a professional practice model that is responsive to the essential requirements of the patients, the staff, and the organization.

Ensure appropriate allocation of resources and equitable, competitive salaries.

Position nurses, therapists, social workers, and chaplains to have a strong voice in issues affecting patient care outcomes.

Provide quality patient care within a cost-effective delivery system.

Lead initiatives that foster diversity of staff and create culturally competent care strategies that support the local and international patients we serve.

CHAPTER 2

Research:
Alarming Data Supports
Nursing Concerns

Research is formalized curiosity. It is poking and prying with a purpose.

—Zora Neale Hurston

The following data is a review of many significant research studies about the nursing shortage. I have included three types of research: clinical, organizational, and financial.

The current nursing shortage is different from prior nursing shortages experienced from time to time.

Nurses have been complaining about short staffing for a long time. Studies undertaken at the end of the 1990s confirmed what nurses feared the most—there is a strong correlation between the number of patients cared for by each registered nurse and the number of patient complications and deaths. Even one extra patient added to a nurse's assignment severely interferes with patient safety.

Studies about workplace environments show that nurses are routinely ignored and treated with disrespect. Nurses have frequently described how disrespectful behavior has interfered with their ability to fulfill their patient care responsibilities and to enjoy the same level of professional respect as others.

Managers have stated that nurse staffing cuts have been necessary to balance the budget. Yet studies examining the cost of the nursing

19

crisis have shown that the costs of high nursing turnover exceed the cost of maintaining a stable and adequate nursing staff.

CLINICAL RESEARCH

Excerpts follow from the abstract from one of the largest clinical studies about the nursing crisis:

- How the study was done:

  We used administrative data from 1997 for 799 hospitals in 11 states (covering 5,075,969 discharges of medical patients and 1,104,659 discharges of surgical patients) to examine the relation between the amount of care provided by nurses at the hospital and patients' outcomes. We conducted regression analyses in which we controlled for patients' risk of adverse outcomes, differences in the nursing care needed for each hospital's patients, and other variables.

- Conclusions:

  A higher proportion of hours of nursing care provided by registered nurses and a greater number of hours of care by registered nurses per day are associated with better care for hospitalized patients.... "Hospitals," wrote Lewis Thomas in *The Youngest Science*, are "held together, glued together, enabled to function ... by the nurses" (Thomas, 1995).

  As hospitals have responded to financial pressure from Medicare, managed care, and other private payers, registered nurses have become increasingly dissatisfied with the working conditions in hospitals.

  Among medical patients, we found an association between registered-nurse staffing and six outcomes. Both a higher proportion of licensed-nurse care provided by registered nurses ... and more registered-nurse hours per day ... were associated with a shorter length of stay and lower rates of urinary tract infections and upper gastrointestinal bleeding. A higher proportion of registered-nurse-hours ... but not a greater number of registered-nurse-hours per day ... was associated with lower rates of three other adverse outcomes: pneumonia, shock, or cardiac arrest, and failure to rescue.

  Among surgical patients, a higher proportion of registered-nurse-hours ... was associated with a lower rate of urinary tract infection. A greater number of registered-nurse-hours per day . . . was associated with a lower rate of failure to rescue.

A greater number of licensed-nurse-hours per day was associated with a shorter length of stay among medical patients.

Our findings clarify the relation between the level of staffing by nurses and the quality of care. We found consistent evidence of an association between higher levels of staffing by registered nurses and lower rates of adverse outcomes. (Needleman et al., 2002)

According to *The Wall Street Journal*, "A new study shows that inadequate nursing care can cause devastating problems for patients . . . the findings, which come amid a prolonged nursing shortage, suggest that patients should consider how many registered nurses are on hand when choosing a hospital" (Johannes, 2002).

An Institute of Medicine report concluded six years ago that there were not enough data to show that more nurses improve patients' medical outcomes. Today's study, which is based on six million patient records . . . finally provides the proof . . . having a higher proportion of registered nurses in the total nursing-staff mix noticeably improved care. (Johannes, 2002)

A clinical study from Pennsylvania came to the following conclusions:

Aiken and colleagues linked information from nurse surveys, hospital administrative sources, and hospital discharge summaries to examine whether hospital nurse staffing and educational level are associated with differences in the outcomes of surgical patients.

- The investigators used data from 168 non-federal general hospitals in Pennsylvania, surveys of 10,184 nurses, and information from 232,342 general, orthopedic, and vascular surgery patients.
- After adjusting for many hospital and patient factors, nurse staffing was associated with significant increases in 30-day mortality and failure to rescue. The results suggest that every additional patient in a nurse's workload increases the odds of patient mortality by 7%.
- The investigators estimate that the risk of death was 14% higher in hospitals where the nurse's average workload was 6 patients or more, and 31% higher in hospitals with workloads of 8 patients or more, compared to hospitals where nurses cared for 4 or fewer patients.

- A direct comparison of staffing hospitals uniformly at 8 vs. 4 patients per nurse yielded estimates of 5 excess deaths per 1,000 patients, and 18 excess deaths per 12,000 patients with complications.
- Having found an association between nurse staffing and patient outcomes, the investigators analyzed whether other nurse characteristics, such as years of experience or educational level, are associated with mortality rates. . . .
- Nurses' educational level was strongly associated with mortality. The authors estimate that the odds of 30-day mortality and failure to rescue would be 19% lower in hospitals where 60% of the nurses had bachelor's or higher degrees than in hospitals where only 20% of nurses did.
- The results imply that, all else being equal, substantial decreases in mortality rates could result from increasing registered nurse staffing . . . the results . . . suggest that the focus on reducing nurse workloads is a credible approach to improving patient care. (Aiken, Clarke, Silber, & Sloane, 2003).

The Institute of Medicine's (IOM) report, *Keeping Patients Safe: Transforming the Work Environment of Nurses*, took a critical look at the working conditions for nurses in America's hospitals.

The nation's 2.2 million registered nurses (RNs), 700,000 licensed practical and vocational nurses, and 2.3 million nursing assistants constitute 54 percent of all health care providers. Nurses are the health professionals who interact most frequently with patients in all settings, and their actions—such as ongoing monitoring of patients' health status—are directly related to better patient outcomes. Studies show that increased infections, bleeding, and cardiac and respiratory failure are associated with inadequate numbers of nurses. Nurses also defend against medical errors. For example, a study in two hospitals found that nurses intercepted 86 percent of medication errors before they reached patients.

. . . Despite the growing body of evidence that better nursing staff levels result in safer patient care, nurses in some health care facilities may be overburdened. For instance, some hospital nurses may be assigned up to 12 patients per shift. Available methods for achieving safer staffing levels—such as authorizing nursing staff to halt admissions to their units when staffing is inadequate for safe patient care—are not employed uniformly by either hospitals or nursing homes. (IOM, 2004)

ORGANIZATIONAL RESEARCH

Nurses have been unable to improve their workplace because they do not have enough power. Many organizations have dismissed

nursing concerns and censured nurse reporters. This has reduced the nurses' willingness to keep trying to make improvements.
Consider the following common situations.

- A nurse tries to reduce wasteful bureaucracy, but no one pays attention to his concerns.
- A patient is injured because his nurse's attempts to eliminate a safety hazard are ignored.
- A nurse feels constant frustration when she must face the same problems day after day.

Researchers at Harvard Business School examined these issues and came up with the following results.

> We propose that how employees respond to problems encountered on the job is a critical factor in enabling or preventing positive organizational change.... Our analysis of quantitative data suggests that problem-solving behavior of frontline workers may reduce an organization's ability to detect underlying causes of recurring problems and thus take corrective action.
>
> ... The first author observed 22 nurses in eight different hospitals for a total of 197 hours. She made observations on all three shifts and on all days of the week.... In 197 hours of observation of 22 nurses, we documented 120 problems (or approximately one every 1.6 hours of observation). Examples include the following.
>
> 1. Missing or incorrect information
> 2. Missing or broken equipment
> 3. Waiting for a resource
> 4. Missing or incorrect medication
>
> Missing or incorrect information, the most time consuming type of problem, included not having a Tylenol order to treat a patient's fever, looking for test results, and not being told about a patient's nausea during a change-of-shift report. (Tucker et al., 2002)

Discover the reasons why health care organizations aren't learning from their mistakes. We are repeating the same mistakes over and over again, a most wasteful and unsafe practice.

First-Order Problem Solving

When nurses encounter problems in their jobs, they essentially have two choices: solve only the immediate problem, or solve the root cause as well as the immediate problem.

Consider the first choice, fixing only the immediate problem. This is called first-order problem solving. If a nurse runs out of a supply of towels, for example, they can be borrowed from someone else. This solves the immediate problem, but does nothing to eliminate the cause. It also may create a problem for somebody else, because the department where the towels came from may then run out of towels.

Second-Order Problem Solving

Another choice in problem solving is to identify and eliminate the root cause as well. In other words, in addition to getting more towels, you find out why you ran out of towels in the first place. It is called second-order problem solving when you diagnose and alter the underlying cause of the problem to prevent recurrence and improve performance.

Why Is This Study Important?

The nurses in this study used first-order problem solving most of the time. This means that their problems were likely to recur because the cause was never eliminated.

This study indicates that work environment is a critical factor in the success of clinical nurses. Organizations are failing to improve because nurses are unable to use second-order problem solving. Nurses have to face the same problems happening over and over again without much chance to intervene. It's no wonder that nurses burn out.

According to the study, health care work environments actually fostered first-order problem solving. The study found that there are three specific aspects of work environments that prevent nurses from engaging in second-order problem solving.

- Nurses have too little time to resolve the problems.
- They lack effective communication channels with people who can help.
- They have lower status relative to doctors and administrators. (Tucker et al., 2002)

I have seen managers, just like clinical nurses, who often use first order problem solving. They try to solve staffing problems with higher salaries, sign-on bonuses and other short-term strategies. Many health care organizations are just like the nurse who borrowed the towels and never learned why there was a shortage. Organizations poach nurses from others without using second-order problem solving to diagnose the underlying cause of why their nurses left.

The good news is that these environmental factors are within our control and can be changed. Change may not come easily, but it is easier than enticing disenfranchised nurses to return to what has become an unsatisfactory work environment.

Implications about Safety and Quality

The towel example was a minor problem. However, this study also uncovered the potential for larger mistakes (Tucker et al., 2002).

During the study, an OB nurse had a consistent problem, finding that infant security tags had fallen off on several occasions. Because the purpose of those security tags is to prevent infant abduction, the potential consequences were serious.

Another example of situations with serious consequences was uncorrected medication mix-ups, which can easily cause patient harm. Consider some similar situations from my own experience, examples of nurses having difficulty with their environment: Nurses without easy access to information about medications that are too new to be in the reference books are unable to follow the safe practice of being knowledgeable about the medications they administer; or nurses who miss early indications of patient complications because their time is so consumed by lesser tasks.

Think about your own experiences. Review your organization's incidents and consider whether they could have been avoided if your culture and working environment had been different.

Ideas for Positive Change

- Encourage nurses to use second-order problem solving to find the root causes of the problems.
- If you are the manager, be a good role model.

- Eliminate the root causes of your own problems.
- If you are a clinical nurse, keep track of recurring problems and provide the necessary feedback for your organization.

A general rule of thumb for change is to address psychological, organizational, and institutional factors together.

FINANCIAL RESEARCH

The nursing shortage has resulted in a vicious cycle of cost escalation because nurse turnover includes many hidden costs. For example, organizations must spend money on advertising, interviewing, and training new staff. They many need to budget for premium pay in order to staff their facility during transition periods. New staff members are usually less productive at first, and this also costs money.

Consider the following cost estimates of nurse turnover from the Nursing Executive Center:

Typically the accounting cost of nurse turnover per nurse is $10,800. However, that number only represents 24% of the real cost. The hidden costs, productivity costs that represent 76% of the true costs, raise the total turnover figure to $42,000.

The number is higher for specialty nurses. Here the typical accounting figure of nurse turnover for specialty nurses is $11,520. Adding the hidden costs makes the total cost for specialty nurse turnover $64,000.

A 500-bed hospital can save $800,000 per year if they reduce their nurse turnover from 13% a year to 10% a year, a mere 3%. (Assumptions: 500 bed hospital; 500 FTE RNs, composition of turnover: 60% med/surg RNs, 40% specialty RNs). (Nursing Executive Center, 2000)

A December 2003 article in the Toronto Star stated that the "employment picture [was] grim for Ontario nurses." It went on to say that "Ontarians are poised to lose about 9,878 registered nurses aged 50 or over. . . . The province must move aggressively to retain experienced registered nurses." The article then discusses the implications of the nursing crisis on the SARS outbreak.

The Australian Patient Safety Foundation via *The Australian* (January 2004) states the following:

Australian Patient Safety foundation president, Bill Runciman, says that many errors by medical staff are caused by a combination of factors, and that the continuing shortage of doctors, nurses and hospital beds only serve to compound any original problem.

The research data about the nursing crisis is riveting. With so many research studies and such large patient populations included in the studies, this research gives great validity to what nurses have been saying for many years.

The fact that these issues have continued for so long, and that nurses have not been taken seriously in their own right, says so much about the work that needs to be done to improve health care by improving the way we treat nurses.

Read on. And, read on with a solution frame of mind. Smart Nursing has many constructive suggestions from which to choose.

Part II

The Six Building Blocks of Smart Nursing

CHAPTER 3

Respect: Learn to Value Nurses

It is part of the healthy instinctual psyche to have deep reactions to disrespect.

—Clarissa Pinkola Estes

Many physicians and managers have become respectful of nurses. Consider these examples:

- A physician collaborates with nurses and together they tirelessly respond to the needs of a critically injured patient
- A nurse, contacting a physician-on-call about her concern for a patient, receives a timely and appreciative return call
- A physician reviews the assessments of an observant nurse and modifies the patient's treatment plan
- A manager warmly expresses sincere gratitude to her hardworking nursing staff
- A physician builds a warm working relationship with the nursing staff

Why do these efforts go unrecognized?
But imagine if you were a nurse in the following situations:

- You enforce a hospital-wide safety protocol and receive irate responses from physicians who feel inconvenienced.
- You report a negative response to a physician's prescribed treatment and find yourself on the receiving end of his wrath.

- You have an excellent work record but have been targeted for disrespect by your manager's ill temper.
- You are working near a highly stressed physician who takes her irritability out on you.
- You make several suggestions to solve a patient safety problem, only to be ignored by your manager. After a patient is injured, action is finally taken.
- You ask to "read-back" a physician's order to reduce medical errors, but the physician refuses to listen.

If you were the nurse in these situations, wouldn't you feel resentful? Physicians and managers who exhibit this kind of behavior are small in number but their influence is widespread.Their actions are damaging, and they discount nurses' valuable contributions. Disrespectful behavior toward nurses results in medical errors, chaos, and a generalized decline in quality of care.

> *Disrespectful behavior directed toward nurses results in medical errors, chaos, and a generalized decline in quality of care.*

Recent surveys indicate that patients respect nurses highly.

Nurses once again scored the highest in an annual Gallup poll of Americans rating the honesty and ethical standards of people in various professions. Nurses topped the ranking of 23 professions in the Nov. 2003 poll, with 83% of respondents rating them "very high" or "high" for honesty and ethics, up from 79% last year. (AHA News, 2003)

Although organizations, managers, and physicians usually use respectful words when describing nurses, their actions often reveal the opposite.

Nurses are censured when they have complaints about management or physician directives. Prior to the current crisis, many managers summarily dismissed outspoken nurses and sought to hire more submissive ones.

*The Color of Fear** was a three-part seminar addressing the nature of racism. The course features a video in which minority males discuss their personal experiences with racism.

———————

*Available at stirfryseminars.com.

I responded to the discussion in ways that puzzled me. I identified strongly with the men's feelings, and asked, "Why do I, a white American female, feel so much like the minority men in the video?" The minister leading the course, familiar with the experiences of nurses working in negative cultures, replied, "It's because oppression feels the same, no matter what the cause."

> *"Oppression feels the same no matter what the cause."*

The oppression of nurses darkens health care. As a nurse, I struggle to respond to that oppression.

People often react unthinkingly to negativity with more negativity. But that response achieves little. Therefore, I have attempted to respond to health care negativity with many positive solutions.

Gary Zukav, in his book *The Seat of the Soul*, likens evil to darkness. He said that we can't eliminate darkness with more darkness. We can only remove it with light. Similarly, we can only replace disrespect by developing respect (Zukav, 1990).

Employers who treat nurses with disrespect have eroded nurse self-respect. They delude themselves when they expect nurses to be productive working under such conditions. What they don't realize is that the most accurate and productive nurses are the ones with the most self-respect.

Who is responsible for the disrespect of nurses? The answer is: physicians and managers.

Although they are in the minority, a substantial number of physicians and managers do engage in disrespectful behavior and verbal abuse directed toward nurses. Because the offenders repeat their behavior many times a day in many facilities around the world, these attitudes spread.

Some progressive managers are actively curbing disrespect for nurses with sanctions. A few have even gone as far as filing complaints to the medical board. As a result some physicians have had to change their behavior or lose their medical licenses. But all too frequently, the abusive behavior continues. It would be a nice change if the managers and physicians who are guilty of nurse disrespect would voluntarily become respectful.

The physicians and managers involved have exploited nurse powerlessness. Many times nurses are treated even worse if they complain. Unfortunately, most respectful physicians and managers consistently look the other way, and do not police their own. This reluctance to intervene turns many health care centers into epicenters of harm instead of centers for healing. As a result, many ill-treated but caring nurses have left health care for other employment.

Trust is necessary for patient safety, nurse recruitment, and teamwork. When nurses trust physicians and managers, they feel comfortable being autonomous. This enables them to be fully engaged in caring for patients without having to waste time wondering if they will be supported. This raises nurse productivity the right way and enables your organization to be financially viable.

How do you build trust? You build trust by respecting yourself and others. You build it by being a role model, by courteous communication, by sensitivity to the needs of others. Staff members pay attention when you seek them out and ask for their input. They trust you when you are consistent and when you make decisions according to what is right rather than what is easy.

Abraham Maslow developed his hierarchy of needs in 1954 when his book *Motivation and Personality* was first published (Maslow, 1954). Nurses and other health care professionals have used this philosophy to understand patient behavior, but don't usually think of it as affecting themselves.

Take a fresh look at Maslow's hierarchy to consider how it can help you to understand the nursing crisis.

Maslow developed a concept that distinguished five levels of human needs ranging from basic, lower order needs to social and psychological needs of a higher order. As you may remember, people need to have their lower order needs met first before they can focus on higher order needs.

Consider how we use this hierarchy in patient care. Patients who struggle with obtaining their basic needs for food and shelter may not be able to concentrate on higher level needs such as health teaching.

Applying Maslow to nursing, consider nurses who transfer patients from their beds to their chairs with too few staff. It is a frequent cause of serious back injury, a violation of basic physical needs.

Or what about nurse Jones who arrives at work to find that only three licensed staff are working instead of the usual five. She is told, "We'll do what we can to help you." Nurse Jones is scared and angry. She is scared that she will miss treatable complications or make a serious medical error. She is angry because so many previous nurses have resigned due to multiple understaffing situations. Management has violated nurse Jones's basic need for safety and security.

Are you ignoring Maslow's hierarchy of needs relative to nurses? Consider common complaints: understaffing, unsatisfactory work environments, and mandatory overtime.

How can you improve nurse recruitment and retention using Maslow's concepts?

Physical: Nurses thrive in Maslow-conscious environments because they are supported. They are proud of their patient care and are more productive. They have more energy and the necessary patience for their very demanding work.

The nurses on each unit work together so that each nurse will be able to take necessary lunch and rest breaks. If necessary, the manager rearranges staff to enable everyone to have necessary downtime during busy days (which is usually every day).

Safety: In a Maslow-conscious environment, nurses flourish because they are supported by safety-conscious organizations. Positive outcomes of reduced errors are your reward for supporting patient safety.

Social: Nurses feel appreciated in a Maslow-conscious environment. Their organizations resonate with a spirit of friendliness and warm support.

The nurses within a home-care team plan to get together for lunch several times a week. They find that talking with their peers assists them in providing better patient care. And they enjoy the social interaction and warm support as well. Their manager schedules them sensibly so that they will be able to continue their lunchtime meetings.

Self-esteem: Nurses feel validated in a Maslow-conscious environment, because their organizations view them as autonomous professionals.

A nurse discovers that a patient needs extensive diabetic teaching. He designs an individual plan that starts this patient along the road to true recovery. His manager supports his critical thinking, and encourages him to add to his ability to skillfully manage patient care with innovative approaches.

Self-actualization: Health care organizations find substantial nursing value in Maslow-conscious environments. Self-actualized nurses set their organizations apart from the competition. These nurses innovate, outline improved work practices, and influence other staff members to function at peak performance.

An oncology nurse has developed several nonmedication techniques to reduce pain and stress. She outlines her ideas and teaches the successful strategies to others by publishing her findings.

Patients notice the difference, and your reputation grows. When exceptional professionals want to work for your organization, you achieve a critical mass of excellence that drives your success. Consider becoming Maslow-conscious to improve quality, productivity, and recruitment and retention.

TYPES OF DISRESPECT

Lack of respect for nurses includes both active and passive types. *Active disrespectful behavior* includes blatant verbal abuse. For example, a physician whose patient is in physical decline yells at the patient's nurse. The nurse only pointed out the patient's symptoms, and may even have been the astute one, the one to notice the patient's symptoms first.

As often is the case, the nurse used excellent judgment and skill, only to be degraded by a physician who may or may not have been the cause of the decline.

Passive disrespectful behavior involves disregarding nurse input. For example, a nurse contacts a physician when she or he sees symptoms of a potential complication. The physician ignores the warning. Many times the nurse calls again and again with progressively more severe symptoms, only to be ignored repeatedly.

Like physicians, experienced nurses are very skilled at noticing when patients start going into physical decline. You might call it intuition, but this skill is honed by many years of experience and education.

During nursing seminars, I often ask nurses if they have picked up important patient problems early by using their intuition. Most of the hands immediately go up, and the nurses are able to cite many examples of how their intuition has benefited patients.

Smart physicians pay attention to the intuition of nurses because it raises the safety and quality of their care.

Planning for reasonable assignments is also a respectful manage-ment action. It shows that you value what nurses can and cannot do safely. It shows that you care enough about nurses that you want to care for them both physically and emotionally.

Nurses lose a sense of safety when fatigue increases their medical error rate. For example, giving 50 or more medications after having already worked all night is a recipe for disaster. When mandatory overtime is carried to its extreme, nurses lose so much social life and experience so much fatigue that they can't maintain even a minimal life balance.

Tired nurses cannot respond well to patient needs. You should maximize nurses' ability to do their job well because quality patient care determines your reputation and profitability.

Respect for nurses has been missing in nursing's health care his-tory. This lack of respect for nurses has been a serious mistake. Now that the disrespect problem is out in the open, it is time to call a halt to this behavior. It is time for nurses to practice zero tolerance for disrespectful behavior. And it is time for those who have been disrespectful to learn from their mistakes and immediately stop behaving in this manner.

PROMOTING RESPECT OF NURSES

Tips for Clinical Nurses

- Maintain your self-respect
- Build alliances
- Learn to negotiate well
- Support respectful behavior
- Reduce negativity over past events

(continued)

Tips for Managers

- Promptly deal with issues of disrespect
- Build trust
- Show appreciation
- Do what's right, not just what's easy
- Support your nurses

Tips for Educators

- Discuss respect issue
- Teach assertiveness skills
- Be a role model
- Discuss respect with clinical staff
- Role play potential challenging situations

CHAPTER 4

Simplicity: Focus on the Basics

Waste thrives on complexity; effectiveness requires simplicity.

—Richard Koch

Simplicity involves rethinking our priorities and returning to basic values of trust, respect, and common sense. It is different from oversimplification, which is the desire to find simple solutions for complex problems.

Patient safety should be our most important goal. Some of the keys to patient safety are hiring the right people, hiring enough of them, and providing an environment where they can use their full professional capacity.

Whom should you hire? Hire nurses who are able to think critically, have strong personal and professional values, and exhibit excellent interpersonal skills. Then give them the freedom to determine the best way to satisfy your clients using their best professional judgment.

Health care is not the only industry that has stifled autonomous professionals. Analysis of NASA's Challenger tragedy has revealed that professional engineers, who were the most knowledgeable about O-rings, had warned NASA about O-ring failures at low temperatures, but they were ignored.

Nurses have been warning their organizations about unsafe staffing for years, but they too have been ignored.

Remember, caring people, not policies and procedures, determine whether patients receive quality health-care services.

Complexity has interfered with safety and quality patient care. It causes medical errors, contributes to the nursing shortage, and reduces productivity. Simplification enables staff to remove this obstacle.

William Jessee describes the dangers of complexity this way:

> Frustration with the administrative complexity of the U.S. healthcare system has reached a fever pitch. Patients, payers, physicians and policymakers agree on at least one thing: the complexity costs big money but does nothing to improve patient care . . . [money] and medical opportunity—is wasted in a system that bases a bewildering array of clinical guidelines, diseases management protocols, specialist referral requirements, drug formularies and other aspects of patient care on which health plan the patient is enrolled in, rather than on scientific evidence of what works best . . . the current duplicative, costly redundant system is harming the nation's health. It's time for a change. (Jessee, 2003)

Complexity is unsafe because excessively detailed safety standards rarely match patient situations. Policies and procedures are important, but they are only as good as the people who carry them out. The best way to use your policies is to rely on the judgment of professional nurses as they implement them in a thoughtful way. Our increasingly diverse patient population will continue to raise the need for professionals who know how to think critically.

In his book, *The 80/20 Principle, The Secret of Achieving More with Less*, Richard Koch addresses "cost reduction through simplicity" this way:

> There is a natural tendency for business, like life in general, to become overly complex. . . . They [organizations] do not focus on what they should be doing. They should be adding value to their customers and potential customers . . .
>
> It follows that any organization always has great potential for cost reduction and for delivering better value to customers: by simplifying what it does and by eliminating low or negative-value activities . . .
>
> Major improvements are always possible, by doing things differently and doing less. (Koch, 1998, p. 94)

These remarks are based on the Pareto Principle first identified by Italian economist Vilfredo Pareto (1848–1923). This principle demonstrates that 20% of one's resources will account for approximately

80% of the results. Sales managers use this idea to identify their top sales people, whereby 20% of their sales force is usually responsible for 80% of the sales. (You can even apply it humorously in our weight-conscious society by saying, "Twenty percent of our food is responsible for 80% of our weight gain.") Working smarter, not harder, is another way to summarize the Pareto Principle.

This idea can be used in business to set priorities. For example, Elizabeth, a nurse manager, might ask herself, "Which 20% of my actions will produce 80% of my desired results?" The following five choices might enable Elizabeth to achieve her goals of excellence and efficiency:

- Spending time solving the root causes of problems
- Hiring competent staff
- Responding to patient and staffing issues promptly
- Consistently practicing ethical behaviors
- Focusing on patient needs

Practicing these principles enables organizations to focus on the future. Cindy, a clinical nurse, might ask herself the same questions that Elizabeth asked. How can she maximize her time to achieve the best results?

- Use her intuition about patient symptoms, and intervene early
- Limit her work hours so that she is able to feel well rested
- Use a flexible approach when responding to patient requests
- Communicate with compassion and respect
- Collaborate with others to raise productivity without fatigue

The Pareto Principle is similar to the concept of leverage. A lever is a simple machine that allows you to multiply your results. If you are a gardener, you might use a crowbar as a lever to lift a heavy rock out of your garden. Without the crowbar, the rock would have been too heavy.

When you use the Pareto Principle you can expect the following outcomes:

- Increased flexibility results in customized medical care.
- Faster decision-making highlights the value of autonomous nurses.

- High levels of employee and client satisfaction build organizational success.

Smart Nursing strategies enable you to leverage scarce health care resources, and to do more with less. The foundations of quality care—respect, simplicity, flexibility, integrity, culture, and communication—are all building blocks for efficiency and excellence.

Using Smart Nursing strategies requires you to make some trade-offs, and to give up some things (slay some sacred cows?). Are you willing to make the following trade-offs?

- Give up micromanagement and choose delegation.
- Give up instant gratification and choose long-term results.
- Give up what is easy and choose what is right.
- Give up control and choose staff autonomy.
- Give up rigidity and choose flexibility.
- Give up talking and choose listening.
- Give up judging and choose empathy.
- Give up victimization and choose accountability.
- Give up ego and choose teamwork.
- Give up punishment and choose education.
- Give up coercion and choose negotiation.
- Give up the status quo and choose innovation.
- Give up arrogance and choose humility.
- Give up carelessness and choose safety.
- Give up stress and choose humor.

The next step of simplification is to focus on what is most important to you.

Since health care organizations have many pressing needs, a team approach will enable you to work on several important projects at once. Having a diverse staff will enable you to match up people with the projects that interest them. Some ideas for projects are:

- Eliminating carelessness and promoting safety
- Promoting autonomy and assertive communication
- Understanding what it takes for staff to put their heart and soul in their work
- Planning informal social events

- Transforming waste into something on your wish list, for example, save $5,000 on wasted supplies and use it for unit education
- Reduce duplication and increase direct time with patients

BECOME A BOUNDARYLESS ORGANIZATION

Organizations need some boundaries to function in an organized manner, but health care organizations are allowing their boundaries to wall themselves off from their staff.

One of our most destructive boundaries is the authoritarian boundary. Health care's command and control atmosphere has blocked communication, innovation, and relationships. We have paid a high price: medical errors, high staff turnover, and financial insolvency.

These boundaries have sabotaged staff's pride in a job well done. We need nurse pride, LNA pride, and housekeeping pride. Every health care staff member is equally important. Do you realize that clinical staff are often judged by how clean you keep your facility? This is yet another example of the importance of valuing every employee, no matter what his or her responsibilities are.

Boundaryless organizations represent simplicity because they use common sense as a guide to making decisions. Jack Welch, in his book *Jack* (2001), shared this experience about removing boundaries. His executives needed computer coaching, and Generation X employees, who grew up with computers, were the experts. Welch authorized the Generation Xers to become computer coaches for his executives despite the fact that the executives had higher status positions. He used common sense and matched up those who knew a skill with those who needed to know it, simplicity in action.

Health care executives should be learning about clinical issues from their nurses. How else can you satisfy your customers? Don't you need to know what your customers are saying? Astute nurses will give you the right information if you are willing to listen to them.

Ideas for Implementation

1. Make time to reflect.
   Staff need to make time to reflect about how to work smarter, not just harder.

2. Document intelligently.

    Many times nurses must document the same information in four or even five places. Sometimes this duplication is necessary for legal reasons, but much of it can be eliminated.

3. Adopt zero-based planning.

    Years ago, there was a popular concept called zero-based budgeting. The idea behind it was to start writing a budget with a zero in every column, and then justify the necessity of each entry. This prevented grandfathering in everything from the last year, without quantifying its value. We can do the same with policies and procedures; justify every bit of complexity to be sure that it is necessary.

4. Keep your mind open to new ideas.

    One nurse in the 1980s took a trip to Disney World, and was impressed by their customer service. She asked to use a modified version in health care, but management couldn't see any value. Now, 20 years later, many health care organizations want to learn about Disney's version of customer service.

    Another example: After readmitting a patient, a nurse realized that the patient needed readmission only because of his inadequate discharge planning. To remedy the situation, she and some peers designed a pilot program to improve patient discharge planning. When management did not support them, many of the nurses involved resigned. It is ironic that what they had requested is now the gold standard for discharge planning.

Ask yourself this question: What ideas are we now rejecting that will become the gold standard for 2020?

Health care could have prevented unnecessary complexity, but it didn't. What we need to do now is identify unnecessary complexity and start disassembling it. It is time to simplify, simplify, simplify, and tear down harmful barriers.

PROMOTING SIMPLICITY

Tips for Clinical Nurses

- Pay attention to unnecessary complexity
- Look for simpler ways to do your work
- Praise success stories of simplicity
- Take time to reflect
- Share knowledge with others

Tips for Managers

- Give your nurses autonomy to simplify problem solving
- Seek out root causes of problems
- Talk with managers from other industries
- Use leverage
- Walk your talk

Tips for Educators

- Add decision-making strategies to your curriculum
- Teach simplification
- Discuss occupational barriers
- Simplify your curriculum
- Encourage students to reflect on their work

CHAPTER 5

Flexibility: Be Adaptable

It is not necessary to change. Survival is not mandatory.

—W. Edwards Deming

Managers frequently lament that they need nurses who think critically, yet they fail to understand that nurses need the right environment to be able to be good critical thinkers. The use of critical thinking implies that the organization has the flexibility to change as circumstances do.

Nurses hesitate to make the independent decisions that are required by critical thinking because they have been reprimanded for doing so in the past. They have learned to hedge when faced with choices because their experiences have taught them that hedging is safer than taking a stand. This ingrained habit is difficult to break. The best way to change this situation is to support your clinical nurses consistently, coach them to make better decisions, and celebrate their successes with them.

Are policies, procedures, and protocols important? YES! But policies are black-and-white, and patient needs come in shades of gray. That is why we need competent professionals. We need nurses with good judgment and critical thinking skills to apply organizational policies to patient needs in a way that makes sense.

CRITICAL-THINKING SKILLS

How Managers Can Encourage the Critical Thinking of Clinical Nurses

- Make your nurses feel *safe* when being decisive. Always support them. Delegate decision-making authority along with responsibility.
- Coach your nurses so that they can tweak their decision-making skills. Sit down with staff members periodically, review their recent decisions, and guide them to become even better decision-makers.
- Substitute positive feedback for censure. Clinical nurses who are sure of their manager's support outperform other nurses.

Why don't nurses say yes to patients more often? Nurses feel safe when they can say, "I followed policy to the letter," even if patient needs remain unmet.

How Clinical Nurses Can Cultivate Critical-Thinking Skills

- Ask yourself, Is this patient request illegal, unethical, or harmful? If not, find a way to fulfill most requests to a patient's satisfaction.
- Put yourself in the patient's place. Ask yourself, What is motivating this patient? Why is it important to this patient?
- Instead of saying no, find a way to say yes. When patients ask for something, listen fully, and give them what they want if at all possible.
- Use your creativity. Innovate and start new patient-satisfaction trends.

FLEXIBILITY

Rigidity Is Expensive

Rigidity wastes nursing time. Rigid protocols are hurdles for nurses to clear before they can focus on patient needs. Autonomous nurses who satisfy patients' needs with flexibility save time and raise patient satisfaction. Multiply these small segments of time saved by the number of nurses in your facility and then by their salary. The financial savings add up quickly.

Rigidity interferes with patient satisfaction. Patients dislike waiting to have their needs met. Rigidity blocks patient safety because it prevents nurses from taking quick action to solve urgent problems.

Patient Dissatisfaction

Bureaucracy sabotages individual effort. Many health care systems merged during the last 10 years in order to survive, forming integrated networks composed of hospitals, physician practices, medical specialty groups, home care, and satellite hospitals.

This strategy has been the opposite of what non-health-care businesses have done, which is to become smaller, decentralized, and "leaner and meaner." This has made them more flexible and able to respond quickly to shifting market demand.

> *It is more important than ever for nurses to be autonomous and able to make patient care decisions at the patient level.*

The Patient's Perspective

First Scenario

Mr. Jones, a patient who is 100 pounds overweight, has been put on a 1,000 calorie weight-reduction diet during his stay at a long-term-care facility until his leg ulcers heal. He receives one half of a hamburger, a few vegetables and pieces of fruit, and black coffee for lunch. Mr. Jones's resentment about his dietary restrictions and lack of dietary control builds every day. Will this dietary regime provide any long-term benefit for Mr. Jones? Hardly. Mr. Jones will probably eat even more when his stay in the long-term facility is over. Good luck to Mr. Jones.

Second Scenario

Nurse Smith understands how to make a real difference with Mr. Jones. She asks his doctor to order a regular diet, enabling him to make his own food choices. She, along with the dietician, works with Mr. Jones to learn how to make better food choices. She asks the food service to provide Mr. Jones with high-bulk, low-calorie foods such as stir-fries and vegetable soups. She reminds him how weight reduction can improve his quality of life and enable him to return to his hobby of fly-fishing. Motivation, flexibility, and patient involvement make a big difference to Mr. Jones, who continues to gradually lose weight after discharge.

In the first scenario, the staff required Mr. Jones to follow a rigid, senseless plan. In the second, nurse Smith thought critically and used a flexible approach. Although Mr. Jones was not able to lose a dramatic amount of weight immediately, nurse Smith's thoughtful intervention started him on the road to healthier living.

Flexibility Strengthens Medical Ethics

Organizations often think that their rigidity is the best way to provide ethical care, but that is not so. Read what Marvin T. Brown says in his book, *Working Ethics* (1990):

> *People . . . interested in ethics will understand the differences be-tween an* ethics of rules, *which attempts to* control *behavior, and an* ethics of decision making, *which* empowers *people and organizations.*
>
> —Marvin T. Brown

Staff empowerment is again considered to be vital for effective management. Consider how this concept can be applied to the nursing crisis. A charge nurse discovers that a patient is in physical decline. She reports the patient's deteriorating condition to the physician who fails to grasp the severity of the situation. The charge nurse also takes her ethical responsibility to her patient seriously and confers with the supervisor. Supervisors generally choose one of two options: (a) They do what is easy. If they fear offending the physician, they play it safe and fail to act, which leaves nurses without any support while they advocate for patients. Or (b) supervisors do what is right. Great supervisors choose the second option and do what is right despite potential criticism.

Consider this example of doing what is right: After a supervisor conferred with a charge nurse about a patient's deteriorating condition, she called the physician back herself. Although the physician lived 30 minutes away and it was 10:30 at night, he arrived at the hospital to examine the patient within 45 minutes.

This illustrates the ethics of decision-making that empowers people. The supervisor, as an empowered manager, intervened appropriately to promote the patient's best interest.

Consider the following example about the need for flexibility as reported by W. Mitchell (1997), a paraplegic patient who was undergoing rehabilitation. He had already recovered from severe burns from a prior accident.

> I had to fight mighty battles for privileges that are taken for granted in the real world . . . For example, there was the battle of the telephone system. When this second accident had occurred, I was quite a successful businessman with interests and investments all across the nation. On a normal day, I made perhaps thirty telephone calls, and I had no intention of changing that. The insistence on rest and quiet in hospitals is often just an invitation for the patient to worry about his awful fate. I chose to get on with my life.
>
> The hospital's telephone system required every call to go through an overworked operator, and it shut down completely at 8 p.m. It was adequate for chatting with one's wife about how the kids are doing in school. It was a disaster for someone with needs like mine. . . . I actually became the first patient in the history of that hospital to have a private, outside line strung into my room at my request, and at my expense, of course. (Mitchell, 1997, p. 63)

Mitchell's long-term goal in his chart was probably something like the following: Achieve maximum physical and mental functioning.

Following hospital policy to the letter and denying Mitchell the phone line sabotaged this goal and would have *decreased* his mental and physical functioning, the opposite of his plan. Was his request illegal, unethical, or harmful? No!

Consider how a lack of critical thinking would have interfered with Mitchell's recovery had he not insisted in having his needs met:

- It would have reduced his rehabilitation potential.
- It would have disrupted his relationship with the treatment team.
- It would have compromised his ability to function as a success-ful businessman.

Times Are Changing

Complex health conditions demand flexibility. Our increasingly di-verse population and 24/7 culture has created an expectation of flexibility among our patients.

Our nursing role will become more advisory and less regulatory in the future.

The Internet has enabled patients to collect abundant data, but it does not help them acquire the skills needed to interpret this information, or to use it to make smart decisions.

Escalating medical error rates have influenced staff to become even more rigid and to follow policies to the letter.

> *The rigidity of the ethics of rules has become another root cause for errors, because it leaves no room for professional judgment as in the ethics of decision making.*

Clinical Nurses and Staffing Flexibility

Sally arrives for work at 11:00 at night. She hears that the supervisor has been unable to replace two nurses who have "called in." *Sally wishes that she had called in too.* Then she would have been able to avoid this problem. Sally knows that she will be expected to manage a much larger assignment. But she also knows that the patient acuity is very high, and if she accepts too heavy an assignment, she risks making serious errors.

Although Sally wants to be a team player, she knows that this kind of situation happens frequently, resulting in a vicious cycle of nurses burning out and seeking other careers. Sally knows that if she is too flexible, management will not solve the root causes of the staffing problems, and she will end up enabling a dysfunctional system to continue.

A Manager's Perspective on Staffing Flexibility

Your job as a manager involves scheduling adequate staff and ensuring patient safety. Because short patient stays result in large numbers of unplanned admissions and discharges, unit acuity can shift dramatically hour by hour. It makes no sense to be overstaffed on one unit and understaffed on another. But the nurses complain every time you ask them to float to another unit. You think to yourself, *"Can't the nurses be a little more flexible?"*

THE ROOT CAUSES OF INFLEXIBILITY

Obsolete Power Structures

Many health care organizations have remained autocratic, and their centralized command and control structures are slow and ineffective.

Successful organizations consider frontline workers to be the most important because they are the ones who interact directly with customers. It is well documented in the literature that many thriving companies owe their success to expert utilization of frontline staff.

Obsolete power structures cause organizations to sacrifice three important goals: customer satisfaction, profitability, and productivity.

Exploitation

As members of one of the helping professions, many nurses report that their profession has deepened their generous nature. As a result, they often feel obliged to work extra hours so that patient care doesn't suffer. They feel substantial guilt thinking that patient needs will go unmet if they don't volunteer to work extra shifts.

A certain amount of generosity is commendable, but nurses burn out when managers constantly ask them to relinquish their free time to fill staffing holes. With fewer nurses, the vicious burnout cycle goes round and round.

Consider the following example of the exploitation of nurses' generous natures:

A nurse answered an ad from a staffing agency and arranged an interview. Although the agency was in another state, the ad had stated that they were looking for a New Hampshire nurse to fill a particular contract. When the nurse arrived, she introduced herself. No one said hello; they didn't introduce themselves; they didn't even describe the work. One said to the other, "This is the New Hampshire nurse." They gave her an application, showed her where to sit, and asked her to fill out the application.

Naturally, the nurse asked a few questions. First, she asked about the nature of the work, and then about the salary. When they quoted the salary, they quoted a rate of pay that was only 50% of the usual rate for that area. When she questioned the manager about the low salary, he replied, "Well, the nurses do it to help out." It was an egregious exploitation of nurses' generous natures.

Discomfort With Ambiguity

Our environment is becoming more ambiguous, and nurses will need greater self-confidence in their ability to make smart choices. A nurse may ask, "Should I go on for a graduate degree?" If so, which one? Since everyone needs to pick their battles in life, nurses will need to decide whether a particular work problem is important enough to take a stand or if they should go with the flow. If they decide to take a stand, they will need to choose the best way to be effective. And they will also need to decide if they are willing to accept the potential consequences.

Fear of the Unknown

Change does feel uncomfortable at first, and people are more likely to make a few errors when they learn new skills. For example, learning to write for publication is often slow in the beginning, but rapidly accelerates with regular practice. However, comfort zones eventually become more like jails when people consistently refuse to accept new experiences and opportunities. Since health care changes rapidly, nurses who refuse to change may find that their job opportunities are greatly reduced because their skills no longer match patient needs.

Peer Pressure

People need support to work in challenging environments. If support for flexibility and critical thinking is absent, nurses become cynical, rigid, and reluctant to trust management. Staff band together and close their minds to new management initiatives.

SOLUTIONS

Create a Culture of Appreciation

Low morale is inevitable when nurses are continuously understaffed, work in disrespectful environments, or are censured for speaking up. Solutions to these issues are challenging, but resolution is definitely management's responsibility.

- Say thank you.
- Wheel and deal. For instance, "If you will work on Thursday, I will give you the 3-day weekend off."
- Offer time off during less busy times.

Sample conversation:
    Manager: Since we have a high census tonight, we will need an extra nurse tomorrow. I know it is your day off. Is there any chance that you could work tomorrow and take a different day off this week? I would really appreciate it.
    Clinical nurse: Well, I have Saturday off, and taking Friday off too would be nice. How about giving me Friday off instead?

Manager: OK. Sharon wants to work on Fridays so she can take your place. Thanks for being so flexible.

Create Flexibility

A multigenerational workforce requires flexibility. We have four generations of nurses working side by side: Matures, Baby Boomers, Generation Xers, and Generation Ys. Generational differences are potential sources of conflict, but not when we value what each brings to the table.

The Matures (or traditionalists), born between 1900 and 1945, number about 75 million people. The Baby Boomers (1946–1964) are at 80 million. Generation Xers (1965–1980) number 46 million, and Generation Ys (or the Millennials) are at 76 million (Lancaster, 2002).

Consider what we can learn from Generation X, who are thought to have the following attributes:

- They want independence.
- They value a satisfactory work/life balance.
- They desire self-development opportunities.

Reflecting on the past, Mature generation nurses, also called the silent generation, were too silent about disrespectful behavior and our lack of autonomy. They have left a legacy of caring, but also one of powerlessness.

It is easy to see why health care cultures can be mismatches for Generation X nurses. Traditional top-down management styles discourage nurses from being independent and accountable. Frequent use of mandatory overtime prevents nurses from maintaining a healthy work/life balance. Moreover, we expect nurses to sacrifice their own needs for the good of the organization.

The effect on patient safety can be illustrated as follows: An 11–7 nurse with an excellent safety record is required to work mandatory overtime, 16 hours from 11 p.m. until 3 p.m. She administers the morning medications, as required, and makes two serious medication errors, most likely caused by fatigue. The patients are harmed, and the nurse is harmed too, because she can't maintain her personal safety standards. Angry patients, dissatisfied nurses, and expensive litigation damage the organization.

Give Independence

When managers and physicians support accountability, nurses can function as frontline risk managers because clinical nurses have the most patient contact and see potential risks early. Attract Generation X nurses by offering professional autonomy. Other industries value Generation Xers' entrepreneurial attitude. We should too.

Encourage a Healthy Work/Life Balance

A healthy work/life balance for clinical nurses also promotes patient safety. Nurses want a life as well as a living. Retention increases when you offer nurses a challenging career that doesn't consume all of their energy. Having energetic, rested employees results in higher safety levels and higher profitability.

Offer Self-development Opportunities

Promote an entrepreneurial attitude. Assign nurses to work on patient safety projects. Empower, coach and support them. Capitalize on Generation X's interest in self-development. Involve nurses from other generations; cross-train them. Everybody wins when employees become lifelong learners and increase their skill level.

Consumers need flexibility due to their diverse needs. Autonomous caregivers are better able to meet those needs, and patients enjoy the benefit of nurses who function as advocates.

Flexibility reduces medical costs. Trying to save money with rigid policies only drives costs up. Flexibility is what satisfies patient needs and saves money in the long term. Patients are often satisfied with less expensive alternatives that rigid policies often exclude. Flexibility reduces waste because customized care enables patients to receive only the specific services that they need.

Case managers are good examples of how customization reduces cost. The financial savings of using case managers far outweigh the cost of their salary.

For example, a patient who is entitled to receive personal care by a licensed nurse's aide really only needs a housekeeping aide or companion aide. The case manager approves payment for the less expensive housekeeping aide.

As another example, a patient is entitled to spend time in a rehabilitation center, but the patient is willing to substitute less expensive home care. You save money while still satisfying patients.

It is time for health care organizations to respond to our rapid changes in society and technology and to be more flexible. We need employees who are able to respond to an increasingly diverse patient population. We need flexible people who can use our constantly changing array of medical technology. We need flexible nurses and managers who know how to motivate their diverse staff to work together.

PROMOTING FLEXIBILITY

Tips for Clinical Nurses

- Use common sense
- Work toward high patient satisfaction
- Innovate
- Become partners with management
- Manage stress with a sense of humor

Tips for Managers

- Support staff's critical thinking
- Be flexible yourself
- Decrease the waste of unnecessary complexity
- Reduce bureaucracy
- Expect your nurses to make decisions at the patient level

(continued)

Tips for Educators

- Encourage students to think for themselves
- Talk about the power of innovation
- Develop nurses' critical-thinking skills
- Be a flexible instructor
- Become educated about health care economics

CHAPTER 6

Integrity:
The Foundation
of Ethical Practice

Integrity is not just a noble idea, it's a tool for personal and corporate success.

—Gay Hendricks

Are you faced with the dilemma of maintaining your integrity while constantly adapting to change? Many times, it's hard to know what to change and what to preserve. Sometimes it takes a crisis to differentiate between those who choose honesty as a core value and others who think of integrity as merely a public relations convenience.

Integrity empowers you. Integrity is an antidote to chaos because it increases self-respect. High self-respect creates order in your life because it is the one constant that you can depend on when everything around you is in turmoil.

Integrity has practical advantages because it saves you time and energy. In his book *The Road Less Traveled*, M. Scott Peck explains the value of honesty this way:

> [People] don't have to construct new lies to cover old ones. They need waste no effort covering tracks or maintaining disguises. And ultimately they find that the energy required for the self discipline of honesty is far less than the energy required for secretiveness. (Peck, 1978, p. 63)

59

In *The Millionaire Mind*, author Thomas J. Stanley interviewed 733 self-made millionaires and asked them to rate their most important secrets to success. Honesty was rated number one (Stanley, 2000, p. 34).

Integrity is a sign of strength. Weak people and failing organizations are the ones most likely to resort to unscrupulous actions. When weak people realize that their inadequate abilities don't measure up and that they can't succeed by being smart enough, they try to achieve their goals using dishonesty (see Figure 6.1).

10 HABITS TO DEVELOP INTEGRITY

1. *Remain committed to integrity.* Some like the idea of integrity but discard it during tough times. Others can maintain their integrity through even the most turbulent times. Why? Because they

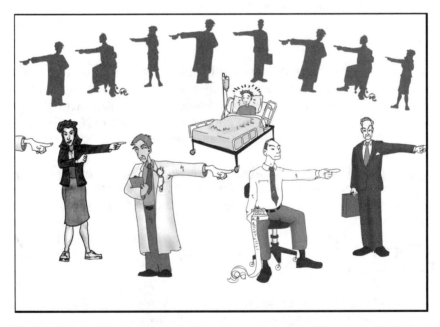

FIGURE 6.1 "Look, they're blaming each other! They wouldn't turn their backs on me if they had to wear a 'Johnnie' like I do."

have adopted effective habits. These habits enable you to thrive, not just survive during chaotic times.

2. *Pick your battles.* Focus on what is important. We live in a diverse society, which means that others behave according to many different styles. Without adequate understanding, these styles can seem threatening. Learn to differentiate between differences in values and differences in style. With style differences, go with the flow, but stand firm with values conflicts. You will burn out if you allow every minor difference to upset you. Prioritize and decide what issues are most important.

3. *Assess the motivation of others.* If someone behaves in a questionable way, ask yourself if inadequate education is the cause or if there is malicious intent. Suppose someone neglected to report information to a physician. It makes a difference whether the error was an oversight due to poor organizational skills or if the information was deliberately withheld. Each circumstance requires a different response.

4. *Develop patience and persistence.* Be patient and persistent with yourself as well as with others. It takes time for people to change so you will need to have a long-term approach. Two ways to support people undergoing change are (a) giving specific directions and (b) being generous with praise.

5. *Be specific.* Clarify exactly what you would like changed. If you want to change something about yourself, define your goal and create an action plan. If you want other people to change, ask them to summarize your request in their own words to be sure that they understand. Expect some errors at first, and be willing to be a coach.

6. *Use praise.* Remember to praise yourself as well as others. We all enjoy approval. People usually respond to praise by renewing their efforts even with difficult tasks.

7. *Learn multiple styles of response.* Using different approaches for different people is a wise choice. Using multiple styles of response enables you to choose the most appropriate style for each occasion just as you choose different ways to dress for various occasions. Using multiple styles doesn't change your basic identity any more than changing clothes does, and people appreciate the individual attention.

8. *Use your intuition.* Most people have developed extensive intuition by accumulating knowledge and experience. It is your

inner wisdom. Use it. In his book *The Confident Decision-Maker,* Roger Dawson says, "Use logic as a tool, but to be a great decision maker, you must blend in the magic of intuition" (Dawson, 1993, p. 72).

One of his suggestions is to write down five major decisions. First decide if they were good decisions or bad. Then analyze whether you used mainly intuition or logic (Dawson, 1993, p. 28). When I did the exercise, I discovered that my best decisions were mainly intuitive. When you have enough time, it is perfectly acceptable to have an intuitive feeling and put the decision on the back burner to give yourself time to reflect. As time goes on, you can decide whether you made the best decision.

9. *Cultivate a network of good people.* Few people thrive in isolation because most of us need supportive people around us. Spend as much time as possible around other people with integrity. You motivate and support each other and will have a dependable group of people to call upon. It's nice to have a reliable network already in place when new opportunities become available.

10. *Welcome personal and professional growth.* When you have integrity, you become real. You solidify your self-respect, which is the basic ingredient of self-confidence. It grounds you. The consistent thread of integrity throughout all of your activities strengthens everything you do.

Patient choice issues are very fluid. Managed care had severely restricted patient choice when it started; it then briefly became more flexible; now restrictions may return in response to higher costs.

Patient trust is very important, and caregivers need integrity if they expect to earn their patient's trust. Some try to fake integrity, but patients quickly find out the truth and discount your messages. In contrast, patients who work with caregivers they trust build helpful relationships with their caregivers.

Multimillion-dollar deals as well as pressure for profitability beckon you to stray from the integrity path. But, long-term opportunities for profitability disappear when companies fail to value honesty. Your credibility is marred if you fail to act with integrity and deliver adequate customer service.

Most health care professionals prefer working for an organization whose mission matches their own value system. But many have found this to be difficult because so many health care organizations send mixed messages to consumers and health care professionals, making it difficult to determine what their mission really represents.

The news carries messages about organizations that have lost the basic values of honesty and civility as they search for greater profitability. Other facilities follow basic values but are under extreme stress about their survival. They cannot always be faulted. Government agencies and insurance companies often set reimbursement rates lower than the cost of care.

A REFLECTION ON ETHICS

In his book, *Working Ethics* (1990), Marvin T. Brown advocates using ethical reflection to assist in decision making.

> The first and primary condition for ethical reflection is the organization's moral community and the moral life of its members and constituencies. How we live with others, our environment, and ourselves constitutes our moral life . . . (p. 180)

> The independence of ethics comes from the act of reflection—of thinking about our moral response to situations . . . (p. 181)

> Ethical reflection should not be seen as some isolated activity apart from the regular process of making decisions. Instead, ethical reflection belongs within the already established decision-making processes, in dialogue with other types of methods for deciding what should be done . . . (p. 182)

> For ethical reflection to be effective and to actually elicit participation, the process itself must be empowered, which in turn empowers those who engage in it. (p. 182)

Suppose an organization decides to cover up a mistake. They will need to add more fabrications to avoid exposure as time goes on, and their deceit will snowball. Eventually they will spend most of their time and energy covering their tracks. This organization is raising its risk of failure because it has little time and energy left to achieve the positive goals needed for success. Huge cover-ups, Enron style, are a good example of how severe a lapse of integrity can be.

Integrity is always the right choice, and it is easier in the long run. Integrity preserves staff energy and prevents future problems. Your consistent practice of integrity builds staff respect, motivation, and productivity.

PROMOTING INTEGRITY

Tips for Clinical Nurses

- Be consistent
- Pick your battles
- Be persistent
- Use your intuition
- With issues of style, go with the flow. With values issues, stand fast

Tips for Managers

- Use a long term perspective
- Praise examples of integrity
- Hire staff with high integrity
- Build a culture that values integrity
- Encourage staff independence

Tips for Educators

- Include integrity in ethics curriculum
- Include news reports of integrity issues
- Be honest about industry issues to decrease new graduate reality shock
- Keep up your own knowledge of what is being written about integrity and ethics
- Encourage abstract thinking

CHAPTER 7

Culture:
The Art of Creating
a Staff-Friendly Organization

When you combine a culture of discipline with an ethic of entrepreneurship, you get the magical alchemy of great performance.

—Jim Collins

Culture matters. Any group achieving long-term success—whether a work group, a family, or a professional organization—will most likely have a positive culture. Positive cultures support members with personal and professional growth and success.

Consider how one work group promotes the success of its facility:

Patients notice that the staff collaborate and seem to enjoy their work. When one staff member is busy, another one pitches in to help. Confident and autonomous nurses, who address patient needs immediately, ensure patient satisfaction. Many physicians prefer this kind of facility because they want their patients to experience quality, consistency, and individualized care.

Families also enjoy the benefits of positive environments:

Parents and their children enjoy their home as a relaxing sanctuary. They feel it is safe to explore new challenges, secure in the knowledge that they will have support even with failure. Mutual trust enables all of the family members to live up to their full potential.

Notice the way this professional organization enables its members to soar to new heights:

The organization has high standards. It keeps raising the bar and motivates its members to set difficult goals. Veteran members generously support new ones by sharing their expertise. This builds commitment and enables members to contribute to the organization that welcomed them so warmly.

Words that describe positive cultures are supportive, generous, confident, sharing, warm, safe, secure, trusting, excellent, achieving, collaborating.

Negative health care environments interfere with productivity and have become obstacles to nursing excellence. The lack of courtesy and respect chips away at nurses' sense of self, sapping their energy and motivation. This prevents employees from using their full potential.

CEOs drive health care cultures. Consider Frank, CEO of the fictional Expertise Hospital System. He sets the tone for the whole organization. He sincerely respects the work of every employee and exhibits a supportive attitude during staff interactions. He shares power and encourages other managers to follow his lead, to treat employees fairly. This means that the managers encourage staff at all levels to contribute their ideas. Managers feel proud of the way their direct care staff have raised patient satisfaction and reduced medical errors.

Frank has a congenial style and often takes the time for casual conversations with nurses and other staff. Employees have a strong sense of loyalty to him and to the whole organization. As a result, employees are consistently more productive than nearby facilities with negative cultures.

Keeping Patients Safe: Transforming the Work Environment of Nurses, the November 2003 report by the Institute of Medicine (IOM) of the National Academies (2004) focused on the environment where nurses work, and the culture that they experience. The report states in part:

"The health care workforce needs to be substantially transformed to better protect patients from health care errors," says a new report from the Institute of Medicine of the National Academies. The report calls for changes in how nurse staffing levels are established and mandatory limits on nurses' work hours as part of a comprehensive plan to reduce problems that threaten patient safety by strengthening the work environment in four areas: management, workforce deployment, work design, and organizational culture.

. . . "No one or two actions by themselves can keep patients safe," said Donald M. Steinwachs, chair of the committee that wrote the report . . . "Rather, creating work environments that reduce errors and increase patient safety will require fundamental changes in how nurses work, how they are deployed, and how the very culture of the organization understands and acts on safety." (IOM, 2004)

Consider this situation where staff collaborated to prevent errors.

A nurse discovers that a patient's address book has been lost. She is upset about the patient's loss and initiates a brainstorming session with the other team members. They come up with an idea that simplifies the management and labeling of patient belongings. After the change, the charge nurse leaves the following note for the nurse manager: "This was the problem, and this is how we solved it. FYI."

After applying the innovation, there were no lost belongings for more than 2 years, a quality-enhancing and cost-effective result for an hour's worth of work by five people.

The problem was completely solved and needed no follow-up by the nurse manager. These empowered staff members saved significant management time. And the empowered nurses enabled this manager to increase his own productivity. Organizational support of nurse autonomy resulted in high quality care, reduced risk, and effective teamwork.

> *Empowered nurses save management time.*

Magnet hospitals have given a well-needed boost to positive cultures by showing why they are necessary for patient care excellence. They have also promoted nurse autonomy by showcasing results of patient and nurse satisfaction. Nursing leaders from magnet hospitals express the importance of culture this way:

The nurse leaders involved in various research studies reported:

A supportive organization sends its message loud and clear that nurses are its most crucial asset, and that providing excellence in patient care is the most crucial outcome. Good patient care comes from satisfied nurses, and you can't get that order mixed up. (Upenieks, 2003, p. 462)

> *"Good patient care comes from satisfied nurses."*
> —magnet hospital nurse leaders

Organizations that promote nurse satisfaction provide the best patient care, while those with an opposite approach end up draining away employee energy.

Read what Barbara Reinhold, PhD, says about negative cultures in her book, *Toxic Work*: "Toxic work situations sap your energy . . . then the insidious eating away of energy and self-esteem begins in earnest" (Reinhold, 1996, p. 16).

As frontline direct care employees, nurses generate good ideas to make their jobs easier without losing quality. When nurses work in negative cultures, they keep those good ideas to themselves. Organizations are the losers because ideas needed for their survival are lost. Morale declines when nurses realize that they are powerless to act and improve their situation.

Before the nursing shortage, nurses who suggested improvements were met with the following attitude: "If you don't like it here, there's the door. We'll just get another nurse." This attitude influenced nurses to keep their silence to avoid being considered troublemakers. Since the start of the nursing shortage, with fewer nurses to hire, managers became more concerned about nurse turnover. But by then, many nurses had already left the health care industry.

Review the way that the following CEO's expectations cost his facility a significant amount of money.

When asked about nursing turnover, a long-term-care CEO replied, "Oh, we're doing great. We've lowered our nurse turnover rate from 70% to 30% a year."

My answer was "That's certainly a step in the right direction, but do you realize that every time you lose a nurse, you lose about $50,000?" As he multiplied $50,000 by the number of nurses he had recently lost, he replied, "I never thought of it that way."

Clinical nurses are also partly responsible for the high nursing turnover. Many times, nurses undermine others, particularly new nurses. This adolescent style of interaction results in petty jealousies and complaints that drive many nurses from the industry.

Have you ever heard the following comments? "Nurses eat their young." "She couldn't handle it." "He's a space cadet."

Anger, fear, and jealousy are three negative emotions that have become obstacles to nurse collaboration. You lose power when you exhibit negative emotions, and waste energy that could have been used constructively.

Negative cultures prevent consumers from receiving full value for their health care dollar. Lost nurse productivity represents a significant amount of money that could be used to add value to patient care.

Fear, miscommunication, and lack of collaboration are all root causes of medical errors. For example:

- A medication dose doesn't make sense, but the nurse avoids calling for clarification because the physician has a history of angry responses.
- The operating-room staff fail to communicate the sponge count accurately. When the patient fails to heal, an X-ray reveals that a sponge had been left in the body.
- A staff member hesitates to ask for lifting help. The negative environment has conditioned him that asking for help is unacceptable. Both the patient and staff member are injured by the resulting patient fall.

Relationship management is one of the best ways to improve organizational cultures. Smart Nursing builds staff commitment and loyalty by promoting positive interactions with all staff members. It is based on the following principles and assumptions:

1. Leaders and managers are more effective when they build strong relationships with their staff.
2. Organizations that provide environments where nurses can perform at their best attract and retain the best people.
3. Long-term strategies such as effective communication and staff-friendly cultures enable organizations to achieve the best results.

Remember, building relationships is one of the best no-cost strategies to improve health care.

One quality necessary to build solid relationships is a sense of trust.

Think about your own life. Who are the people you trust? What attributes do they have that determine trustworthiness?

Write the numbers 1 to 10 on a piece of paper. List the 10 most important qualities in other people that you think represent their trustworthiness. Those are the qualities to develop within you. Your list may include dependability, sincerity, and a caring attitude. Talk with other people and ask them what is on their list. Then use those qualities as your guides as well. Add the element of time because most people want to evaluate your behavior over a period of time to see how consistent you are.

People are more likely to trust when each side displays a consistent code of ethical behavior. Some people want to improve trust but don't want to make the first move. Trusting makes people vulnerable. If they have been burned in the past they are reluctant to have it happen again.

Both managers and clinical nurses have made mistakes. Management has allowed unsafe staffing, and nurses have had unrealistic expectations. Restoring trust involves cultivating mutual respect. We must honor what each side brings to the table.

The first step in building trust is to scrap your obsolete power structure. All health care professionals are equally important, and everyone should be treated with respect.

Listening is the second step. Listen to others with an open mind and without preconceived ideas to distort what you hear. Review the following list of specific descriptors for trusting relationships between managers and clinical staff.

- Managers and staff value their differences, and view them as assets to use for the patient's benefit.
- Staff and managers work as partners.
- They share the same vision.
- Managers empower their staff.
- Clinical staff and managers are both accountable for results.
- They enjoy mutual respect.
- They produce quality care.
- Managers address errors promptly and seek to discover all of the relevant facts.
- Managers avoid using fear and punishment. They substitute relationships, communication, and education instead.

With trust and good communication, managers are able to start building commitment. Commitment enables you to build a culture where people feel a sense of freedom to "be themselves" as they work together. This kind of freedom enables staff members to use their full professional capacity and to share their knowledge for the good of the whole organization.

An ambulatory care nurse notices specific education needs of a patient in the emergency room. He addresses this need with a customized and comprehensive patient education plan that will prevent future ER visits.

This response would not have been possible if he had worked in a negative culture. Fast paced ER environments leave little time for patient education. An ER nurse may not be able to spend time and energy on important functions such as education when most of his time and energy is consumed by a negative workplace. A negative workplace prevents nurses from accessing their "higher selves," the natural overdrive that people experience when they become engrossed in their work.

Clinical nurses must act as mature professionals. Welcome diverse perspectives and support each other. Ask yourself:

- When was the last time I said thank you to another staff member?
- Do I listen when my peers try to communicate?
- How often do I ask my peers if I can help them complete their assignment?

Participating in a positive culture means using your sense of humor. Humor has the ability to deepen relationships and relieve stress. Think back to times when you shared a good laugh with another. Didn't you feel more relaxed? Haven't you felt stronger relationships with people who make you laugh?

Next time you attend a corporate event, notice which departments are having the most fun. They are usually the ones receiving the most awards because humor promotes productivity and quality.

You can also use humor as a vehicle to deliver negative news. Humor is like a parachute—it gives negative information a soft landing. However, this only happens if you use humor skillfully and with sensitivity.

Humor is like a parachute. It gives negative information a soft landing.

Clinical nurses—Adopt the following ten suggestions to promote a positive culture:

1. Invite new nurses to join you for breaks and meals.
2. Start a new support group for new nurses.
3. Become a preceptor. If you are already a preceptor, take a refresher course to improve your skills.
4. Request the education department to bring new nurses back to vent positive and negative feelings, and improve orientation.
5. Be a good role model for others.
6. Support effort as well as success.
7. Give encouragement when someone tackles a difficult assignment.
8. Collaborate to obtain feedback and improve care. Support other people's projects. Be as enthusiastic about their projects as your own.
9. Increase your own self-respect. How can nurses ask for the respect of others if they don't respect each other? Our self-image influences our treatment of others. When defensive, we perceive situations selectively, and assume that the results will be negative.
10. Cultivate a win-win attitude. Exhibit an attitude of abundance. Encourage your peers to contribute their full potential. When we embrace our differences, we will be able to use everyone's ideas to resolve our health care challenges.

Health care companies need positive organizational cultures, because well-treated employees promote patient satisfaction. For example, managed-care organizations (MCOs) have an opportunity to support strong customer service. This means supporting patients with education and assistance through difficult times.

Health care organizations interact with many groups: patients, families, employees, providers, physicians, the government, and insurance companies. Keeping an open mind, instead of becoming judgmental, enables staff to represent their company as compassionate, knowledgeable, and progressive. A good image is important because it attracts customers. A positive culture is an opportunity to project your best image.

A positive workplace energizes its staff. Now, nurses are draining themselves dry trying to finish all of the work they are assigned as well as surviving a negative environment. Atmospheres on patient units influence how well people recover.

Health care companies administer Medicare and Medicaid programs with mixed reviews. More government involvement in managed health care is a strong possibility. Whether this trend continues depends on how well facilities resolve their present challenges. Without better outcomes, Americans may prefer to have a single, non-profit agency administer health care. Private MCOs may find reduced demand for their services. They may have to fight for their survival unless they improve their results.

LEARNING ORGANIZATIONS

Every employee in your organization is more important than ever. This means that organizations must consider the collective knowledge of their employees as an asset to be maximized. Peter Senge discusses this concept fully in his book, *The Fifth Discipline: The Art and Practice of the Learning Organization.*

> *It's just not possible any longer to figure it out from the top and have everyone following orders of the grand strategist.*
> —Peter Senge

Senge also points out the importance of *systems thinking.* Systems thinking is focused on the "wholeness" of situations. As mentioned in the introduction, both nursing process and Smart Nursing strategies are based on general systems theory, which focuses on the wholeness of situations as well. The systems within which we live are not linear but very complex arrangements. Listen to how Peter Senge uses weather as an analogy to describe systems thinking, and then describes how we can apply systems thinking in our own lives.

A cloud masses, the sky darkens, leaves twist upward, and we know it will rain. We also know that after the storm, the runoff will feed into groundwater miles away, and the sky will grow clear by tomorrow. These events are distant in time and space, and yet they are all connected with the same pattern. Each has an influence on the rest, an influence that is usually hidden from view. You can only understand the system of the rainstorm by contemplating the whole.

Business and other human endeavors are also systems. They, too, are bound by invisible fabrics of interrelated actions, which often take years to play out their effects on each other. We focus on snapshots of isolated parts of the system, and wonder why our deepest problems never get solved. Systems thinking is a conceptual framework, a body of knowledge and group of tools that has been developed over the past fifty years. They make full patterns clearer. This helps us see how to change them effectively. (Senge, 1990, pp. 6–7)

The Benefits of Learning Organizations

Systems thinking is congruent with Smart Nursing strategies, and magnet hospital principles. And it is responsible for the many achievements that successful companies enjoy.

Systems thinking promotes

- trust
- good employee communication
- solid relationships between staff members
- cultivation of diverse points of view
- sharing of power and information

Health care also needs systems thinking if we want to solve our many challenges. Involve your clinical nurses if you want to implement these concepts. Put employee suggestions into effect immediately. If an employee makes a suggestion in a staff meeting, implement it right after the meeting. If that is not feasible, implement it as soon as possible. Your prompt response shows employees that their ideas are valuable. Encouraging employees to think for themselves serves a twofold purpose: You stimulate innovation, and you increase staff satisfaction.

The causes of the nursing crisis began many years ago. The lack of respect has been around a long time, and so has understaffing. But other factors such as the increased complexity of patient care and changes in the role of women in society added to the problem until a tipping point was reached. Around 1995, the nursing problems finally accumulated to the point that nurses started leaving health care. Because these events were distant in time and space, it took quite a few years for managers to understand the whole pattern. And until they could see the whole picture, they were unable to find effective solutions.

It is time for health care organizations to pay more attention to their workplace environments. Even if you hire the best people, those employees will not be able to give you the desired results without a supportive environment. Make the most of your employees' efforts. They are your most important resource. Create a staff-friendly culture.

PROMOTING A STAFF-FRIENDLY CULTURE

Tips for Clinical Nurses

- Maintain a positive attitude
- Contribute your ideas at work
- Support your peers
- Value your nursing contributions
- Teach others to treat you with respect

Tips for Managers

- Be knowledgeable about group dynamics
- Support cooperation
- Put nurse innovations into effect within 24 hours or ASAP
- Create a positive environment
- Recognize that nurses are high-value human resources

Tips for Educators

- Assess your students' potentials and seek to fulfill them
- Provide an open learning environment
- Be knowledgeable about collaboration
- Show students how culture affects nursing care
- Collaborate with clinical nurses and managers

CHAPTER 8

Communication:
A Key Ingredient of Collaboration

The most important thing in communication is to hear what isn't being said.

—Peter Drucker

Communication is an art. As with any art, different people have different styles. Effective communicators continuously scan their own communication patterns as well as those of others. They ask themselves, Are my communication strategies working? If the answer is no, good communicators modify their strategies to fit a new environment.

A variety of individual communication styles can become one of our greatest assets. This communication patchwork reveals the beauty of individual designs, shades, and textures that produce rich communication nuances.

Communication involves many variables—it's not just what you say, but how you say it. And your communication success can also be determined by what you don't say. Because many communication variables are intangible, everyone can stand to develop more communication expertise.

ROLE OF COMMUNICATION ON NURSE RECRUITMENT AND RETENTION

Even a small amount of insincerity on the part of management negates many of their tangible offerings, such as premium pay and bonuses.

How Is Communication Like Romance?

Perhaps one way to view the complexities of communication is by comparing communication to romance—another common life experience that could also be considered an art.

How would you answer the following 10 questions? (Note that I have answered some of the following questions for myself. Your answers may be different.)

1. Are there any hard and fast rules for romance? No
2. Does romance depend mostly on relationships? Yes
3. Is every romance different? Yes
4. Does the fact that you sent flowers or candy necessarily ensure a successful romance? No
5. Can a small amount of insincerity undo a large quantity of tangible offerings (candy and flowers)? Yes
6. Should even small amounts of abusive behavior be enough to end the relationship? Yes
7. Is consistency important? Yes
8. Can you improve your romantic skills by learning from your failures as well as your successes? Yes
9. Is romance an art? Yes
10. Is romance worth the effort? You have to decide that one for yourself.

If your employees view you as insincere, it really doesn't matter what else you do. Insincerity leads to a lack of credibility, resulting in your communication efforts being ignored. In other words, sincerity and credibility are a necessary foundation for your communication efforts. Without this strong foundation, your communications will crumble even if you follow otherwise good techniques.

All health care professionals need to be effective communicators. Nurses complain to each other in coffee breaks, but rarely to managers who have the power to respond to those complaints.

Nurses have gained center stage because of the nursing crisis. Rising to this challenge will require activation of dormant abilities such as curiosity, but the rewards are great—respect, influence, professional fulfillment.

Managers, who have denied the severity of the nursing shortage in the past, must now pay attention to nursing perspectives. They cannot ignore the nursing crisis anymore because it has interfered with the management of their facilities. Now is the time for clinical nurses and managers to brush up on their communication skills and voice their opinions.

COMMUNICATION SKILLS FOR NURSES

Most nurses are skilled with informal nurse-patient communication, but may need to expand their repertoire of some or all of the following skills.

Assertiveness

Assertiveness is an important part of effective communication. In the past, managers often disciplined assertive nurses. But now you can use the nursing shortage as leverage to ask for what you need. Discard negativity, be assertive, and state your needs in a positive way.

Here are some suggestions for becoming more assertive:

- Intervene in situations calmly and confidently.
- Respond to problems in a timely way to avoid accumulation of negative feelings. Those who are passive for a long time run the risk of overreaction to small incidents.
- Clearly articulate the importance of using nursing perspectives.
- Use language that management understands.

"I" statements are important when communicating your thoughts and feelings. But when persuading others to accept your viewpoint, "you" statements often work better because they describe the benefits for the other side.

For example, you could say, "I don't like this policy and I don't think that many other nurses will like it either."

But it would be better to say, "Using this policy will result in the loss of at least three nurses costing you over $150,000." Or, "This change will increase medical errors, drive patients away, and lower your accreditation score." You will be more likely to be successful.

Small Talk

Skill with small talk is an important strength. It builds rapport so that your messages become more effective. Shy people often have difficulty engaging in small talk. But it is a learned skill, and you will improve if you are willing to make the effort.

Improve your small talk expertise:

- Read books on small talk such as *What Do I Say Next?* by Susan Roane (1997).
- Prepare for small talk by reading magazines and newspapers and choosing a few topics to bring up.
- Prepare a few questions that will stimulate other people to talk. For instance, ask people open-ended questions about common topics such as favorite vacations, books, and hobbies. These questions will give you clues about the other person's interests, enabling you to follow up with more specific questions that will continue the conversation.

Public Speaking

Solid public-speaking skills will empower you and make you more visible in your organization. It is a good antidote to the powerlessness of nurses. It allows you to influence many people at the same time.

Consider the following example of an employee who enjoyed a rapid rise to a high management position:

Amy was a supervisor who recognized the value of becoming an excellent public speaker. She joined Toastmasters where she had the opportunity to practice her public speaking skills. She also gained experience as the master of ceremonies for meetings.

Amy used her skills to develop an effective training program for her employees. Her manager recognized her initiative and praised her employees' excellence. Amy's manager had planned to emcee a retirement party for a high-level manager, but was called away by a serious family illness. She asked Amy to take her place at the last minute, because she knew that Amy was an experienced public speaker.

Amy had an opportunity to showcase her communication skills in front of most of the senior managers of the company. Shortly after Amy's successful performance as an emcee, she was given the opportunity to expand her management skills by rotating to several key corporate positions. After her positive performance in these positions, Amy received a promotion to an important high-level management position.

Writing for Publication

Writing is another learnable skill that gives you the opportunity to influence many people with one effort.

One way to learn how to write for publication is to join a writers group (most areas have local writers groups).

What happens when you attend a writers group? Attendees usually bring copies of their writing to the group. Everyone critiques each other's work. Rewriting your piece based on this critique enables you to improve your writing. Writers groups are also good places to learn about the process of submitting articles for publication.

Whether speaking in public or writing an article, numbers can dramatize issues. Saying that lowering nurse turnover by a mere 3% saves a 300-bed hospital over $500,000 annually is more effective than saying, "You will save money if you lower nurse turnover."

APPLYING COMMUNICATION SKILLS

1.   Break the code of silence. Nurses have an informal code of silence because prior attempts to communicate have resulted in reprisals. Nurses have learned that it is smarter to keep their opinions to themselves in order to retain their jobs. As a result, health care has lost nurses' valuable input.

2.   Earn your staff's trust. Many managers have lost their staff's trust. You need to be reliable and trustworthy when you interact with your staff.

3.   Listen. Another way to improve communication is to simply listen. The advantages of listening are many:

- Listening helps you identify problems.
- Listening exposes feelings—those invaluable but sometimes inconvenient traits that make us truly human. We need to manage our feelings and give them a positive focus instead of having to deny them.
- Listening jump-starts the solution process because answers pop up during candid conversations.
- Listening relieves stress. Bottling up thoughts and feelings only depletes our energy.

Some managers want to hear only good news and deny their problems. That's like having an abnormal X-ray and touching it up to make it look normal. It is difficult to solve a problem unless you understand it.

4.   Avoid punitive attitudes. People can't be effective partners if one side is afraid. Conversations sometimes reveal offensive behavior by powerful people, and it takes a brave and politically savvy organization to resolve these issues fairly.

- Show sincere respect for staff ideas.
- Share your goals.
- Collaborate.

Use Body Language Effectively

Nonverbal communication accounts for more than half of how you communicate, with some estimates going as high as 80% to 90%.

Observe your nurses for nonverbal behavior that indicates they are upset but not talking about their concerns. When nurses must work in a negative environment, they absorb that negativity but try to avoid passing it on to patients. Any human being can absorb only so much negativity without burning out. Therefore, managers should treat nurses the same way they would like their nurses to treat the patients. Nurses are internal customers. Patients are external customers. Both kinds of customers need excellent customer service from management.

Consider your nonverbal communication and how you come across to others. Make any necessary changes.

Use Different Communication Approaches

Ask yourself these questions: Does my staff represent a variety of personality styles and cultural backgrounds? Do I use the same approach for everyone? Is my approach based on *my own* needs?

If you answered yes to these questions, consider using multiple approaches for different people. Start using a variety of communication styles instead of just one. For example, if you know a staff member is gregarious and extroverted with a strong need for approval, connect to that person by giving approval in an enthusiastic manner. A staff member with quiet self-confidence may respond best to a calm, logical and systematic approach.

Managers who use a variety of communication styles improve staff relationships. Solid relationships generate the power to produce exceptional patient results.

ACTIVITIES TO IMPROVE YOUR COMMUNICATION SKILLS

1. Assess your image, and make a list of adjectives that describe you. Ask several associates to make a similar list about you. How do the lists compare?

2. Keep a journal for 30 days about your communications approach and results. Try to spot trends. You can also include comments from other managers and staff when analyzing your pattern.

3. Notice good role models. Observe and listen to how they communicate. You will find good role models in many places—at work, at meetings, in public places.

4. Keep a communication log of your *informal* conversations with nurses for the next 30 days. Record the tone of those conversations. Are they warm and genial? Have you communicated with all shifts? Ask yourself who initiated each conversation, you or the staff member?

5.   Ask yourself if you use informal conversations effectively. Informal conversations serve multiple purposes. They can be used for

- Assessing attitudes
- Developing rapport
- Giving attention
- Discovering needs
- Understanding goals
- Validating feelings
- Providing support
- Giving praise
- Correcting actions
- Fact finding
- Self-disclosure

If you have too few informal conversations with nurses, improve your availability by scheduling nonstructured time to talk with your staff. During conversations with nurses, acknowledge their value beyond clinical functions. Consider taking the following actions if you would like to start using nurses as marketers:

- Start a conversation in a staff meeting about the important role of nursing in your organization's overall success.
- Dedicate a portion of your staff meetings to making a list of your current challenges and brainstorming about the opportunities that lie beyond the challenges.
      An example of an opportunity lying beyond a challenge is the following example describing a missed marketing opportunity by hospitals. The first sub-acute units appeared in the 1990s with a patient population consisting of people who had no place to go: patients not appropriate for home care, long-term care, or acute hospitalization. Independent sub-acute companies provided a less expensive alternative for complex but stable medical/surgical, rehabilitation, and oncology patients. Hospitals eventually created sub-acute or transitional units themselves. However, they could have been first in this market if there had been better communication between CEOs and nurses. Nurses and social workers had experienced frustration for some time trying to find

facilities for these patients. With better communication, hospitals would have recognized this situation as an important marketing opportunity and created sub-acute units sooner.

- Establish a corporate writers group to teach interested nurses to learn how to write for publication.
- Form a corporate Toastmasters club so your staff can become more articulate in oral communication. Or encourage staff to join a local community club.

People don't always realize that communication lessons occur around them every day. Learn to pay attention to the way people communicate in meetings, at home, in grocery stores, and listening to your favorite teenager. The sources are endless.

Miscommunication is often harmful, but it can be humorous as well. I sometimes include a book raffle in my education programs, so I called a bookstore and asked the clerk if they carried *The Wisdom of Teams*. She answered by saying, "Well that's an oxymoron if I've ever heard one." I quickly realized that she must have thought that I had asked for "The Wisdom of *Teens*," and must have had a bad time with her teenager that day.

We both had a good laugh and commiserated about the challenges of raising adolescents. But there was more than a grain of truth in this situation. Many teens can be very wise, and can even be good communication role models for adults because many teens are authentic, empathetic, compassionate, and caring while some adults have replaced these essential qualities with cynicism.

Some communication lessons are available to each person every day, as in the following example:

A group leader wanted to encourage one of her members to volunteer to bring refreshments to the next meeting. When no volunteers were forthcoming, she asked them the following question: "If you *were* going to bring refreshments, what would you bring?" She then asked the group to take a vote on their favorite refreshment choice. We all had a good laugh, and of course someone volunteered to bring refreshments. I quickly added the leader's "If you were . . ." question to my communication toolkit.

NEGOTIATION

Conflict is inevitable whenever a variety of people work together, yet many people fail to realize that conflict can be a positive force.

Conflict is positive when you respect all opinions, and combine all perspectives in innovative ways. Consider what Sy Landau (2001) states in his book, *From Conflict to Creativity: How Resolving Workplace Disagreements Can Inspire Innovation and Productivity.*

> *Without the catalyst of fresh ideas and differing perspectives, change and growth are not possible.*
>
> —Sy Landau

Learning how to negotiate is an important skill for all health care staff. As diversity increases, staff members will need more ways to bring people together instead of driving them apart.

Solid negotiating has eluded nurses because nurse powerlessness has made them hesitant to take a stand. Regardless of their view, others have ignored most nurses.

> *Nurses negotiated using their only bargain chip: They voted with their feet and walked out of health care.*

When nurses tried to express their alarm about unsafe staffing, many managers wrongly assumed that the nursing shortage was just another cyclical event that would quickly pass. This prevented nurses from forming effective relationships with management because the balance of power was skewed in management's favor.

Successful negotiators are skillful relationship builders. They nurture trust. They build bridges and bring people together instead of driving them apart. When you strengthen your clinical staff's negotiation skills, you strengthen your whole organization. The result: You bring nursing's clinical perspectives to management.

Most good sources on negotiation techniques emphasize certain principles:

- Use research to understand the perspective of the other side. For example, management and clinical nurses could understand each other better.

- Ask questions.
- Build relationships.
- Think long-term.
- Have a plan.
- Be patient.
- Think win-win.
- Find common ground.
- Avoid wrong assumptions.

You might want to try some specific suggestions:

1. Pick your battles. Focus on what is most important. Some issues are too minor to bother with. If you divide your energy into minute pieces, you may not be able to achieve your most important goals.

2. Increase the size of the "pie." If your budget is too small, generate more revenue (bake more pies) instead of always decreasing expenses (cutting smaller and smaller pieces of pie).

Consider the following example: Professional organizations need positive cultures too. Many nursing organizations have lost members, reducing their dues income, an important source of revenue. As responsible professionals, they have to balance the budget. But if they only cut member benefits, they will start a vicious cycle of further membership declines. To increase the membership, they will need to give members more benefits so that they can attract new members.

Many of the benefits that professionals seek in their organizations are free or inexpensive.

- networking opportunities
- mentors
- leadership experience
- professional support
- collective action on common problems
- support for innovation
- group purchasing

Use care in how you communicate—how you say something is even more important than what you say. Remember, nonverbal communication accounts for up to 80 or 90% of your communication.

3. Avoid inflammatory words—why destroy your chances for consensus with careless communication?

4. Use the "flinch." When the other side makes a statement, act shocked (exaggerate how shocked you are) and remain silent. Many times the other person will modify his or her position.

5. Let the other side speak first. A common motto is, He who speaks first, loses.

6. Use diffusion. I first experienced diffusion when my firstborn child started nursery school. One teacher, very experienced and loving with her small charges, had a favorite phrase whenever she had to deny a child's request. She would just say, "Tomorrow is another day." Since the children couldn't argue with that statement, they would accept it as an answer and calmly walk away without feeling defeated. That's diffusion—making a statement where everyone has to agree. Using diffusion and making a statement like, "The patients need a variety of caregivers," might bring diverse health care staff together.

Consider how nursing issues could have been resolved years ago by using better negotiation:

- Managers would have done research about the average workplaces in comparison to those in other industries.
- They would have sought out nursing viewpoints in a nonpunitive way.
- They would have built relationships with clinical nurses by showing them professional respect.
- They would have considered the long-term implications of severe staff reduction—the nursing shortage.
- They would have used a plan instead of just a quick fix to get them through the immediate situation.
- They would have had the patience to allow nurses to respond to the crisis by increasing their skills, and using productivity measures that didn't interfere with patient safety.
- They would have supported nurses as strong professionals essential to their organization's success.

Now is a good time to apply some of these negotiation principles. Whether you are a manager or clinical nurse, read some negotiation resources such as Dawson (1995), Dolan (1992), Fisher (1981), and

Shapiro (1998). These are listed in the Recommended Reading section at the end of the book. Pay attention to the successful negotiation techniques that you notice day to day. People are negotiating all around you every day.

- A parent negotiates with his or her child while shopping.
- Leaders bring residents together to improve their community.
- Adult children persuade their elderly parents to make necessary housing and caregiving decisions.

Learn from them. Add their effective practices to your own negotiating toolbox. Knowledge builds flexibility and makes you effective in responding to a variety of circumstances.

We need nurses who can become patient advocates. Clinical nurses who are strong negotiators will be able to obtain necessary resources for patients and their families: safe staffing; equipment; funding for important projects; time for direct care; better indirect care systems such as documentation guidelines; and an ability to be an effective patient advocate.

PROMOTING EFFECTIVE COMMUNICATION

Tips for Clinical Nurses

- Eliminate the code of silence
- Learn to speak and write for publication
- Be assertive in appropriate situations
- Have positive expectations
- Build your small-talk skills

Tips for Managers

- Earn your staff's credibility
- Encourage nurses to network with each other
- Respond to communication problems promptly
- Encourage staff participation
- Raise productivity with good communication

Tips for Educators

- Include communication as a major part of your curriculum
- Teach negotiation skills
- Support the value of speaking in public and writing for publication
- Show students the importance of nonverbal communication
- Use experiential learning experiences

Part III

Applications of Smart Nursing

CHAPTER 9

Staffing:
Recruiting and Retaining
the Best Nurses

---

*No company can change any faster than it can change
the hearts and minds of its people.*

—Robert Frey

STAFFING CHALLENGES

Constant staffing changes prevent organizations from moving forward (see Figure 9.1). Health care managers are so preoccupied with recruitment and retention that there is little time to progress in other areas. They have taken nurse availability for granted for many years. Now many facilities are losing important opportunities. The nursing shortage has forced hospitals and nursing homes to close units and delay launching new services.

One way that organizations try to manage nurses is coercion, but coercion is ineffective. In his book *Primal Leadership*, Daniel Goleman describes how coercion can effect staffing.

The business world is rife with coercive leaders whose negative impact on those they lead has yet to catch up with them
. . . When a major hospital system was losing money, the board hired a new president to turn the business around—and the effect was disas-

93

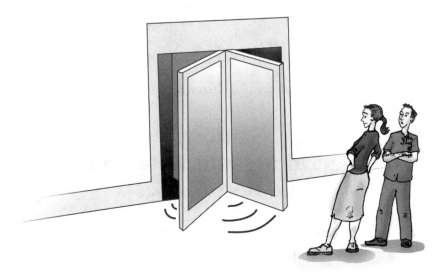

FIGURE 9.1 **"Is this the door to the ER? No, it's the door to HR. The nurses go in and out so fast you can't even see them."**

trous. As one physician told us, "He cut back staff mercilessly, especially in nursing. The hospital looked more profitable, but it was dangerously understaffed. . . . Everyone felt demoralized.

No surprise, then that patient satisfaction ratings plummeted. When the hospital began to lose market share to its competition, the president grudgingly rehired many of the people he'd fired. "But to this day he's never admitted he was much too ruthless . . . " and he continues to manage by threat and intimidation. The nurses are back, but morale is not. Meanwhile, the president complains about patient satisfaction numbers—but fails to see that he's part of the problem. (Goleman, 2002, p. 76)

Unsafe staffing alarms nurses because they are good at recognizing high-risk situations. They know that patient safety suffers from inadequate staffing. Paying attention to nurses reduces risk because nurses notice safety problems in time to prevent catastrophic events.

It is not always necessary to increase staffing. Many times, managers can just rearrange staff to provide better coverage. This practice often causes problems, however, because many nurses oppose floating. Most nurses have been asked to float to unfamiliar units where they feel inadequate.

Many times, nurses have encountered bad experiences such as being floated without adequate preparation where they don't feel clinically competent. Rather than risk their nursing licensure by making errors, nurses simply refuse to float altogether.

Instead of working together to solve mutual problems, managers and clinical staff dig in their heels to form opposing camps. The reason for the lack of collaboration is the distrust that has been built up.

Part of the solution is to use cross-training intelligently. If you want cross-trained nurses, invest your time, energy, and money. Schedule your nurses to work alongside experienced nurses in the new specialty. This means duplicating your staffing, which involves higher short-term costs. You will need to build trust and give cross-trained nurses your support. Tangible incentives such as higher salaries or more vacation time can help, or use intangible rewards such as higher status, participation in desirable projects, or public recognition.

Management benefits from greater staffing flexibility. When the census in one department suddenly changes, you will be prepared to move your staff around without risking patient safety.

MANDATORY OVERTIME

Instead of taking the time necessary to arrange appropriate staffing, many organizations abuse mandatory overtime because it is convenient.

The example here is an 11–7 nurse who discovers that she has been mandated to work 7–3 as well. The nurse loses her need for proper rest, a basic need. Nurses also lose a sense of safety when their fatigue increases their medical error rate. Giving 50 or more medications after having already worked all night is a recipe for disaster. When mandatory overtime is carried to an extreme, nurses lose so much social life and they have so much fatigue that they can't maintain even a minimal life balance.

Most health care organizations spend more than $5 million a year on human resources. In fact, some small organizations invest more than 75% of their budget on human resources.

If you had a personal investment of $5 million in real estate or securities, you would no doubt spend time and energy to increase your return. Why not spend more time and energy reducing human-resource costs?

The nursing shortage has forced facilities to increase their staffing budgets to provide for "premium pay." If nursing coverage with the regular staff is inadequate, organizations end up paying time and a half or double time in order to keep their facility open. Staffing agencies increase costs because their fee includes compensation for both the nurse and the agency.

Earning premium pay may sound like a very profitable arrangement for the nurses, but only in the short term. Nurses cannot sustain excessive mandatory overtime because it is physically and mentally exhausting.

Mandated shifts can also keep them from fulfilling their childcare responsibilities. Consider the following two examples:

At 2:00, a 7–3 shift nurse is told that she has to stay until 11:00. She is a single parent and must pick up her child from daycare at 5:00. This nurse is concerned because she takes her childcare responsibilities seriously. Isn't she exactly the kind of nurse that we must keep in health care? Shouldn't we seek out and support nurses who take their responsibilities seriously? Aren't such nurses also the ones who will take their patient safety responsibilities seriously? When our coercive attitude toward mandatory overtime forces nurses to choose between being a responsible parent and remaining in their profession, isn't something very wrong with a system that requests such a choice? Could this coercive attitude also be contributing to our escalating rate of medical errors?

Another nurse working from 3 to 11 is told she must stay until 7:00 the next morning. She has two preschool children and her husband works during the day, so she must now go all day without sleep until her husband comes home from work at 5:00. After working for 16 hours at a very demanding job, she must go without the rest that she needs.

Both of these nurses are likely to have high rates of illness and absenteeism and will eventually burn out. The short-term gain produced by premium pay quickly evaporates, and many of these nurses will ultimately leave health care for another occupation, deepening the nursing crisis.

REVERSING NEGATIVE SITUATIONS

The nursing shortage is only a symptom. The real issue is that nurses are unable to improve their situation and are worn out from mandatory overtime and unrealistic staffing ratios. These conditions decrease morale and erode nursing spirit.

Health care organizations tend to react to crises instead of acting before problems get out of control. Some spend large amounts of money to recruit and train new nurses but spend little to keep them. Others try to prevent turnover but spend their money in the wrong ways—recruitment and retention bonuses and advertisements. More money doesn't help if nurses feel ashamed of the care they give, if no matter how hard they work or what they do, their professional effort isn't enough.

Senior managers, some with little on no clinical perspective, often create policies that nurses cannot follow in good conscience because they contradict sound nursing practice.

Inadequate Staffing

What happens when an organization cuts staffing without considering the consequences? Nurses, RNs and LPNs alike, then have responsibility without voice. They have too little time to maintain even minimal safety standards, and mistakes happen. Nurses become concerned that they will miss important symptoms because there is little time for adequate observation or follow-up.

Nonclinical people look at patient statistics in isolation. Nurses must look at the faces behind those numbers every day. One of those faces belongs to Sarah.

Sarah is a resident of a long-term care facility. She is frail, a shadow of the vibrant woman she once was. You think about how much she is like your grandmother, whom you would want cared for with safety, with dignity, and with love. As you look Sarah in the eyes every day, you know that there is too little time to give her proper care.

You are a long-term care nurse. You would like to match the caring attitude of Sarah's family.

You start to give morning medications to your 35 residents. You expect to finish your medication pass in about 2 hours, which gives you less than $3^1/2$ minutes per person, not counting interruptions. In that $3^1/2$ minutes, you must wash your hands, identify the patient, position the patient, correctly choose an average of 10 medications, crush those medications, and mix them with applesauce. As you administer those medications, you notice that Sarah only takes about a quarter of a teaspoon at a time. She also has 4 ounces of a nutritional supplement to drink. She only drinks a small sip at a time— about a half teaspoon—and then rests a second or two.

You can do the math; it would take 10 to 15 minutes to administer just the supplement. Facilities are penalized on accreditation reviews if their residents lose weight. Ordering supplements without providing enough time for the staff to administer them is an example of how facilities achieve high health care compliance on paper records, coupled with low quality of care in actual practice.

So you do what you can in $3^1/2$ minutes and then go on to the next resident. Physical assessments, assisting the LNAs, talking with staff and families, and telephoning physicians take more time from resident care.

Some facilities use agency or per diem nurses for every shift. Agency and per diem nurses are excellent, but they should fill specific staffing holes, not constitute most of your staff. Consider the result when a facility is entirely staffed with agency nurses. A 3-to-11 agency nurse in a long-term-care facility receives report from an agency nurse at 3 p.m. and gives report to another agency nurse at 11 p.m. All of the necessary tasks are carried out, but the residents don't even have the comfort of a familiar face.

Such situations are as unfair to the agency nurses as they are to the residents. No matter how skilled the nurse, she or he needs to know something about each resident. How can an agency nurse identify changes in a resident's condition if no one in the facility has any idea about the resident's usual level of functioning? Agency nurses also become disenfranchised when they are unable to deliver high-quality care. Serious errors occur when residents lose their continuity of care.

I received the following e-mail from a long-term-care nurse: "I, too, am experiencing the ravages of too little staff (1–2 LNAs, 1 Nurse: 39 residents) and administration's indifference to our plight. After working for only 6 years as a nurse, I am on the edge of deciding to leave nursing."

A better scenario for long-term care would be what Wilma receives. Wilma is a long-term resident whose son lives locally. However, her two daughters live out of state. Because both daughters are nurses, they manage any medical questions that arise. Staff turnover at Wilma's long-term facility is very low, and the staff function as surrogate family members. When the LNAs pass Wilma's wheelchair, they stop and smile at her, pat her arm, and warmly say, "Wilma, you're looking good today. How are you?" Wilma smiles back. The LPN charge nurse, Sandra, knows both Wilma and her daughters well because she is a long-term employee. She anticipates the kind of information that the family members need to know and calls them periodically. Wilma's daughters are very appreciative that Sandy provides such personalized care and keeps them informed about their mother.

This is long-term care at its best. Low turnover and fair treatment of staff produce quality care for patients and financial viability for the facility. Families want their loved ones to be cared for in facilities such as this, which rarely have any vacant beds.

Unlicensed Staff

Facilities have also tried to save money by decreasing licensed staff. For example, hospitals began hiring unlicensed assistive personnel (UAP) instead of licensed nurses in the 1990s and tended to skimp on necessary training.

Nurses became upset because they were expected to delegate tasks to workers of questionable ability. Delegation laws vary from state to state, but most states hold registered nurses responsible when someone to whom they delegate tasks makes an error.

The nurses had three choices: teach the UAPs how to do the work themselves; perform the tasks themselves (and become more overworked); risk losing their nursing licenses if a UAP made errors.

Nurses expressed their concerns. Few managers paid attention or responded with appropriate action. Many nurses chose a fourth option: They left nursing for other careers. Using UAPs may have been a poor investment.

A 2002 American Nurses Association (ANA) study found that 75% of nurses surveyed said the quality of care had declined in the last 2 years, and more than 4 out of 10 would not want their families to be patients at their facility because of the low-quality care (ANA, 2004).

BUSINESS AS USUAL VERSUS STAFF-FRIENDLY CULTURES

Critical Care in the "Business as Usual" Culture

An ICU nurse describes reporting for work and discovering that instead of his usual one or two patients, he had been assigned four. When he objected, management agreed that it would do what it could to help. Eventually, however, he received a negative comment on his evaluation as a result of his objections.

Critical Care in a Staff-Friendly Culture

Ryan, an ICU nurse, has a two-patient assignment. Because the vents and A-lines require constant monitoring, he is very busy but able to fulfill his assignment with safety and quality. He makes time, for example, to talk with the families of his patients and answer their questions. They appreciate it very much, and Ryan's caring attitude generates a sense of trust. This makes their ordeal of living through a family member's life-threatening illness more bearable.

Home Care in the "Business as Usual" Culture

A home care nurse finds that his increased workload prevents him from taking any morning or afternoon rest breaks. He only has time at lunch to drive through a fast food restaurant and eat while driving back to work.

Finally, after working since 8 a.m., he finds himself filling and programming a narcotic pain-control pump at 7:00 in the evening. Such pumps require exact attention and accuracy because they frequently run for 24 to 60 hours without further nursing examination. In such situations, any small error multiplies with time and can potentially result in a serious injury. The job requires the attention of an alert nurse.

Home Care in a Staff-Friendly Culture

Susan, a home care nurse, has a full morning schedule of patient visits. During her first visit, she discovers that the patient has some medical complications. She is delayed there because after calling the physician, she also has to call an ambulance and remain with the patient until the ambulance arrives to transport the patient to the hospital.

She goes on to her next patient, a hospice patient. She is again delayed. Although this patient doesn't need admission, Susan must call the physician and then perform several treatments that the physician requests.

By this time, Susan is 2 hours behind schedule. However, when she calls her home care office to report the delays, the supervisor lightens her patient load so that she can provide all of the patients with quality care and remain healthy herself. The supervisor knows that one nurse had a cancellation and another had a light patient load that day, so she rearranges the patient assignments. This supervisor knows home care nurses sometimes have unavoidable delays, and she responds effectively to prevent burnout of her staff.

Medical-Surgical Care in a "Business as Usual" Culture

(Note that medical-surgical units now care for acute and complex patients who would have been in the ICU 10 years ago.)

The charge nurse discovers a staff scheduling error at 11:00 p.m. A scheduled staff member who she thought was an RN is in fact a LNA. This scheduling error reduces the unit's licensed staff by one. The oncoming charge nurse feels that another RN is necessary. As she puts it, "We can't even keep everybody alive without another RN." She frantically calls other staff, but none can work. They have already worked too many extra shifts.

She eventually persuades an evening nurse to stay for the night shift. Her reasoning is this: "She can work until she drops." She figures the evening nurse will "drop" at about 5 a.m., so she schedules a day nurse to replace her at that time.

Medical-Surgical Care in a Staff-Friendly Culture

Linda is a medical-surgical nurse on a high-performance team. All of the nurses have substantial patient assignments. Linda notices that one of her patients, Mr. Jones, has suddenly become pale and diaphoretic (sweaty). Although he has a normal blood pressure, his heart rate has increased from 78 to 115. As she assesses him, his vital signs become very unstable, and she calls the cardiac arrest code.

As Linda works with the code team to restabilize Mr. Jones, Kim, another nurse on the unit, responds to the needs of Linda's other patients. All of the staff skillfully fulfill Linda's role until the emergency is over.

Psychiatric Care in a "Business as Usual" Culture

Sally, a psychiatric RN, remarks to Jen, another RN, "Jen, we're working together on Christmas."

Jen replies, "That's great. I love to work with you."

Sally then corrects Jen's perception. "No. You don't understand. It's only *you and I* who are scheduled. No one else."

They both know that six staff members are needed to provide safe care. On Christmas Day, Jen and Sally must get by with a staff equivalent of four: two people working 8 hours with four staff each working 4 hours. No injuries occur, but the quality of care is decreased. And, being two staff short, there was a higher risk of injury for both patients and staff.

Psychiatric Care in a Staff-Friendly Culture

The 3-to-11 staff on a psychiatric unit would like to have opportunities to foster their professional growth by belonging to professional organizations.

Many of the meetings occur in the evening and conflict with the nurses' work time. The evening nurses meet with the nurse manager and create a plan that allows each nurse to choose one organizational meeting they would like to attend. The nurses devise a schedule to cover for each other. They also agree that if a staffing emergency occurs on their meeting day, the affected nurse will volunteer to work and miss his or her meeting that day.

After 1 year, during a meeting to evaluate the results, the staff expresses their gratitude to each other. They have all experienced professional growth in their desired associations. Although they have had to miss an occasional meeting, their job satisfaction is high because they feel valued by their managers and peers.

Organizations lacking a staff-friendly culture fail to realize that negative environments interfere with recruitment and retention That kind of environment diminishes an organization's reputation. Reputation in the community is one of the factors that influence where nurses want to work. Most nurses look at employment ads and immediately eliminate the ones from facilities with poor reputations. Nurses don't apply if they know that the glowing words in the ads are a sham. They may know from talking with other nurses in the community that the facility is severely understaffed, that the care is unsafe, or that they will be treated with disrespect.

SOLUTIONS

Use "Humble Marketing" to Attract Nurses

Nurses, like patients, listen to the buzz about your facility. A positive reputation attracts the best nurses.

Emanuel Rosen says in *The Anatomy of Buzz*:

> 'Humble Marketing' may sound like an oxymoron, but it's not. 'Humble Marketing' occurs when you under-promise and over-deliver, and let the product's reputation spread by itself through invisible networks. When you look at the early days of a product like the Palm computer, which got tremendous word-of-mouth support, you see just that. (p. 13)

Nurses rely on what they hear from their peers when deciding where to work. They ask their peers about safety issues, staff turn-over, and whether they will be treated with respect.

Nurses become skeptical when a facility seems to be replacing most of their staff. If they notice ads for a director of nursing, education director, some supervisory positions, as well as RNs, LPNs and LNAs (all shifts, full- and part-time), they wonder why most of the staff has left. Most good nurses steer clear of such facilities.

Some organizations simply do nothing and hope the nursing crisis will go away by itself. But the revolving door continues to turn with nurses coming and going. Money that could be better spent on acceptable constructive projects goes out of the door with the departing nurses.

View Your Nurses as Assets

Human resource funds are really an investment in your organization. High staff turnover reduces your return on that investment.

Patients consider nurses as essential *assets* to their care, but management tends to consider nursing as an *expense*—a large one.

Good managers are taught to maximize assets and minimize expenses. And because nurses are viewed as an expense, staffing cuts seemed to be a logical way to balance the budget. Indeed, many organizations have cut their nursing budgets severely.

However, those budget cuts have triggered the current nursing shortage and have produced burnout and low morale. In some institutions, the quality of nursing care continues to spiral downward, resulting in a vicious cycle of further revenue shortfalls.

According to generally accepted accounting practices (GAAP), an intangible asset is defined as follows: An asset lacking physical substance. The main intangible used in financial statements is "goodwill" (the monetary value of a business's reputation). (Although GAAP does not allow companies to list expert employees—nurses or highly trained high-tech employees—as intangible assets in financial documents, expert employees still function as assets. They increase a company's value. Therefore, most high-tech companies value their highly trained employees as assets.) And, health care organizations should do the same: Value their nurses as assets.

Document Nursing Value Quantitatively

1. Perform a cost/benefit analysis:
    Managers and clinical nurses can justify their requests with a cost/benefit analysis. For example, Table 9.1 shows how you can quantify the financial advantages of adding one more nurse.
2. Create a ratio:
    In this case, for every $1 that you spend to hire an additional

TABLE 9.1

Cost of adding one full-time equivalent		Benefits of adding one full-time equivalent	
Salary	$51,500	Decreased litigation	$ 500,000
		Avoid premium pay	$10,000
		Decreased sick time	$5,000
TOTAL COSTS	$51,500	TOTAL BENEFITS	$515,000

nurse, you reap $10 in benefits, a sound business decision. Your cost: benefit ratio is 1:10.

3. Calculate your opportunity costs:

You may wonder what the opportunity costs are. Suppose you have $30,000, and decide to buy a car. You could pay $30,000 for your car or you could buy one for $20,000 and have $10,000 left over. If you decide to buy the $30,000 car, by default you give up having a less expensive car with $10,000 left over. The alternative that you gave up represents your opportunity costs. In other words, your trade-off was to give up the $10,000 and less expensive car for the higher priced car.

What could you have done with the $10,000 that you gave up by buying the more expensive car? You could have opened a savings account, gone on an expensive vacation, or used it for a down payment on a house.

Those three items—savings account, vacation, and house—represent part of your opportunity costs. They represent the trade-off that you made: an expensive car instead of something else.

How Do Opportunity Costs Relate to Nursing? Health care organizations have miscalculated their opportunity costs. As described, your opportunity costs are measured by the trade-offs that you make. A common health care trade-off is to save money by using inadequate staffing (short-term solution) and live with the long-term consequences (high turnover).

Another example is that when you allow an unsatisfactory work environment to continue, by default you have chosen high nurse turnover and have given up a stable nursing staff.

(Managers who delay action to repair negative cultures must live with the long-term result, high staff turnover).
4. Calculate the cost of nursing turnover as in Table 9.2.
   As you can see, losing just six nurses costs you $140,000. Your opportunity costs in that situation are that you *could* have spent the $140,000 on giving 50 nurses 2 weeks off with pay or a 2-week education sabbatical for 50 nurses.
   What about the $390,000 it cost you to lose 10 nurses? You could have used that amount on *ALL* OF the following:

   1. A full-time person in charge of solving the root causes of problems ($77,000)
   2. An educational conference for 30 nurses ($15,000)
   3. A college course for two nurses ($3,000)
   4. New computer equipment ($5,000)
   5. Two extra weeks off with pay for 50 nurses, or a 2-week sabbatical for 50 nurses ($140,000)

   You could get *all* of that and still have $150,000 left over.

5. Raise your return on investment (ROI).
   The money you saved by reducing nurse turnover is only the beginning. It gets better. With lower nurse turnover and a staff-friendly culture, quality of care and services improve. Patient safety improves, and risk declines. You avoid expensive litigation that can cost more than $5 million per case.
   High patient safety improves your reputation in the community. More physicians and patients want to use your facility. As competent and experienced nurses become familiar with

TABLE 9.2

Number of nurses leaving per year	6	10*
Cost of orientation	$60,000	$100,000
Cost of premium pay to cover staffing "holes"	$30,000	$70,000
Training associated costs (when productivity is less than 100%)	$30,000	$90,000
Cost of advertising, interview time, sign-on bonus, time to manage short staffing	$20,000	$130,000
Total	**$140,000**	**$390,000**

*Some from ICU and the OR

your excellent reputation, they want to work for you. You become the employer of choice for nurses. You have just turned a vicious cycle of decline into a vitalizing cycle of success. Your gross revenue increases

Plan Your ROI on Nursing

Organizations save money when they decrease nurse turnover. A 300-bed hospital can save roughly $500,000 annually by reducing nurse turnover by a mere 3–5%.

What if you, the manager, could choose the return on your investment? Would you choose 20% or 30% a year? Why stop? Why not double or triple your money? Human resource investments, particularly in nursing, are an investment on which you choose your own rate of return. You only have to act.

For example, assume that as the vice president of patient care you spend $25,000 in a year to educate nurse managers on raising nurse retention: You coach your managers to form solid relationships with their staff (respect each other, act in a trustworthy way, and communicate effectively). You review preferred delegation and decision-making strategies so your nurses can solve patient problems on the spot, without going up and down a long chain of command.

After the training, the managers of 30-bed units are able to reduce their turnover by 3% over the year. Each unit achieves $50,000 savings in recruitment, orientation, and overtime costs. With six nurse managers, you have created a gross savings of $300,000. Subtracting the $25,000 in training costs gives you net savings of $275,000. You have just multiplied your investment of $25,000 in management training costs by 11, to a return of $275,000—*an 1100% rate of return.* You have solidly raised the return on your human resource investment. What a wise choice!

Solve Root Problems

When nurses encounter problems in their jobs, they essentially have two choices: solve only the immediate problem or solve the root cause along with the immediate problem

The nurses in the Harvard University study (Tucker et al., 2002) described in chapter 2 used first-order problem solving most of the time. This means their problems were likely to recur because the cause was never eliminated.

This study indicated that work environment is a critical factor in the success of clinical nurses. What this means to managers is that nurses have to face the same old problems happening over and over again without much chance to intervene. It's no wonder that clinical nurses burn out.

The good news is that these environmental factors are within management control, they are free, and they can be changed easily.

Organizations need managers who are willing to identify and solve root problems. How?

- Think about your own experiences. Review your organization's incidents and consider whether some of them could have been avoided if you had identified their root causes.
- Apply some of the suggestions from the Harvard study:

First, if workers are to engage in root cause removal, this activity must be an explicit part of their job and enough time allocated for removal efforts.

Second, there needs to be frequent opportunities for communicating about problems with individuals who are responsible for supplying front line workers with materials or information. . . . There must be convenient opportunities in the course of the day for workers to give feedback. . . .

Third, when the signal is given that there is a problem, proper attention must be paid to it. We must recognize communication as a valid step in the direction of improvement. Often the best that the worker could do was to merely raise the issue, but too often this worker ran the risk of being considered a "complainer." We did not observe any instances where the nurse contacted someone about a trivial or insignificant exception. In fact, we observed several occasions where we were surprised that the nurse did not raise awareness around a problem that we felt could have serious consequences. (Tucker, 2002)

Review the following positive statement from Dennis O'Leary, M.D., President of the Joint Commission on Accreditation of Healthcare Organizations (JCAHO), who took the following position on health care staffing and safety during his testimony before the Senate Committee on Governmental Affairs in June of 2003.

This country is neglecting to concomitantly improve the professional education system to support the new thinking about prevention of errors and adverse events in this complex delivery system. We need to graduate health care professionals who are proficient in "systems thinking," who are comfortable using decision support tools, and who can actively engage in solving patient safety problems. (JCAHO, 2003)

Both physicians and nurses must work together to solve health care's challenging problems.

RELATIONSHIP MANAGEMENT

Autocratic management styles are still quite common in health care and have contributed to the nursing crisis.

Some organizations have tried to reverse this trend with shared governance. Shared governance recognizes the value of building relationships and listening to nurses. Organizations who use the shared governance model give nurses professional autonomy and hold them accountable for results. You must be willing to share power and avoid micromanaging if you want to implement shared governance. Micromanagement commonly occurs when you delegate responsibilities to another and then oversee every minor detail. Micromanagement is unpleasant for the delegatee, and the duplication of effort wastes time and money. Micromanagement also destroys innovation because the delegatee is prevented from using his or her full professional capacity.

Nurses who have been involved in committees for a number of years have found that their input is often ignored. As a result, they lost interest when their efforts turned out to be just "busy work." This has been an expensive mistake.

Consider the cost of an average committee. Twenty nurses attending meetings for just 1 hour each month costs over $6,000 a year. This wastes a lot of money unless you actually implement the nursing feedback.

Nurses had high expectations when nursing committees first became common in the late 1980s. However, they started becoming cynical when their reasoned input was disregarded. As a result, health care management lost much of its credibility.

Nurses expect sincerity, trust, and good communication from management. For instance

- Discuss your staffing strategies with your nurses to be certain that they understand and are able to support it.

- Give your nurses autonomy. Coach them to be independent instead of asking them to consult with you about every decision.
- Teach your nurses to be good leaders and decision-makers because autonomous nurses save management time and raise patient satisfaction.

Suppose a cardiac patient's family has had a difficult adjustment to his hospitalization, reacting with underlying anger and fear. The charge nurse slowly forms a relationship with the family. They ask her to help them solve a problem they are having with visiting hours. She devises a plan, clarifies the limits, and finalizes a customized plan to meet their needs.

This charge nurse is responsible for three important accomplishments: (1) better customer service; (2) stronger patient loyalty (reduced patient resentment that often leads to litigation); and (3) solving a patient problem without needing management intervention.

When you champion your nurses, you build strong relationships with them. Nurse managers must insist that the staff be respected every time. Good managers enforce the policy, "We don't 'do' rude here," and they support nurses who assertively enforce this philosophy as well.

For example, a physician in a hurry can't find a chart that he needs and makes an irate comment to a nearby nurse. She calmly acknowledges his need for the chart, but is clearly assertive and explains that his angry comment was not appropriate. She says, "I get frustrated looking for charts too, but it's not okay to take out your anger on me."

This nurse knows that her nurse manager will support her even if the physician complains about the limits she set.

Disrespectful behavior is a common problem for nurses. It leads to high nursing turnover unless management maintains a respectful workplace.

Nurses are knowledge workers, and they constitute an important part of your organization's intellectual capital. Now, intellectual capital is considered one of the most important assets within companies. Successful companies are the ones who have learned to use their intellectual capital effectively.

Adequate rest for your staff is an insurance policy for management success. Even equipment—capital assets—need downtime. Think about how much more important your human assets are to your organization's success.

Nurses need time to rest. Review your full-time nurse schedules for the past 6 months, and look for the number of times each nurse has had a 4-day stretch of time off. If your nurses have worked without a minimum of two 4-day breaks in the past 6 months, you are risking staff burnout. Your nurses need enough downtime to recharge their energy.

Assess your responsiveness to nursing needs. Calculate how many staff issues have remained unresolved for 60 days or more. Unresolved issues (frequently unsolved root problems) are one of the major causes of the nursing crisis. Review your unresolved issues, and set a 30-day deadline to resolve them. Create a timeline to measure the steps toward solutions. It may help to create a critical path to keep you on schedule (Table 9.3).

Or, delegate your unresolved issues to the clinical nurses involved, along with enough authority for them to implement their decisions. Then support the decisions that your nurses make. Clinical nurses need managers who are willing to create and maintain positive work

TABLE 9.3 Critical Path

Week 1	Week 2	Week 3	Week 4
Vacation schedule	Talk with staff	Write tentative schedule	Final schedule
Increase charge nurse autonomy especially for staffing and safety responsibilities.	Meet with charge nurses to ask for input.	Meeting to coach charge nurses and discuss staffing strategies.	Meet with charge nurses to begin new responsibilities, to set up communication channels, and to schedule ongoing opportunities for further discussion.

environments. They need managers willing to support them, and they need managers who understand nursing's true value.

Are you up to the challenge?

PROMOTING SMART STAFFING

Tips for Clinical Nurses

- Keep a healthy life/work balance
- Think long term
- Value your work
- Be patient
- Support management's positive staffing efforts

Tips for Managers

- Avoid mandatory overtime
- Use stable staffing to increase patient satisfaction
- Motivate; don't coerce
- Hire for attitude/train for skills
- Utilize the intuition of nurses

Tips for Educators

- Teach students how to be good at coaching
- Include problem-solving strategies in your curriculum
- Be honest about staffing issues
- Maintain your own clinical skills
- Avoid defensiveness

CHAPTER 10

Teamwork:
Building High-Performance Teams

If teams learn, they become a microcosm for learning throughout the organization.

—Peter M. Senge

Use teamwork to address the following health care issues:

- Managers will continue having difficulty staffing their facilities due to increased demand for health care services and decreased supplies of nurses.
- Workloads for nurses and other health care workers will continue to increase.
- Medical errors will continue at a high rate.
- Baby Boomer health-care requirements will raise the demand for additional services. Baby Boomers are educated, articulate, and assertive and will not allow their needs to be put off with weak platitudes.
- The bottom line of many health care organizations will continue running in the red in direct proportion to the high costs of finding and retaining competent staff.
- Organizations will need the efficiency and financial savings that high-performance teams offer.

A serious obstacle to high-performance teams is the attitude of "every nurse for herself." This attitude has proliferated for various

113

reasons. Authoritarian and coercive management styles have resulted in dysfunctional cultures that block cooperative efforts. But nurses themselves have often returned to adolescent behavior styles, focusing on rejection and pitting one staff member against another. Nurses and managers must work together using high-performance teams to rise above these two challenges if they hope to alleviate the nursing crisis.

Nurses need positive cultures and high-performance teams so they can work smarter, not just faster. Instituting high-performance teams costs nothing because the key factor is attitude, of both staff members and management.

In my experience, I have found high-performance teams raise productivity without increasing medical errors or nurse burnout. Since health care is labor-intensive, this higher productivity also reduces costs.

Consider a typical day on a high-performance team:

The nurses arrive for work. They don't object to heavy assignments because they know others will help them if their workload becomes unmanageable. Patient care units are unpredictable because most patients are medically complex and unstable. One nurse caring for five patients may have to manage several medical emergencies at the same time. Staff members can manage these emergencies better when everyone works cooperatively.

High-performance team members value diversity and ask each other for advice. Mutual respect builds commitment to the team and results in everyone's accomplishing more. Everyone pitches in when three admissions arrive during a 2-hour period. While the RN is assessing the patients, the secretary or LNA orients the patients to the unit and the LNA helps the secretary assemble the charts. Later, the secretary may be swamped with orders. The RN notes extra orders or enters them into the computer. They all work as hard as they can, no matter whose job it is.

In the end, the workload evens out fairly. Staff members remember how others helped them when they were the busy ones. They joke with their colleagues to manage stress. As they leave work they say, "I can hardly believe how much we were able to accomplish today." They feel pride and gratitude for the team that helped them to accomplish so much. They were able to accomplish more with less effort.

High-performance teams also prepare units to manage unexpected staffing problems. Consider the following example:

All of the licensed nursing staff on one shift were sick for a week, except one RN and one LPN. The RN was able to manage the unit with less nursing staff by delegating things in a different way. Within legal limitations, certain parts of the admission process and other work usually assigned to nursing staff were delegated to licensed nurses' aides. This certainly was not an optimum situation, but it helped them survive a temporary staffing shortage and gave them flexibility without sacrificing quality.

Is this situation a fantasy? No. This scenario is a composite of the day-to-day experiences of nurses working on high-performance teams. Team members use humor to decrease stress and create a relaxed working environment and positive atmosphere for patients who would sometimes comment, "We love it when the nurses laugh with each other." They are also able to model stress management techniques.

The foundation of high-performance teams is a web of positive relationships built over time. The manager often initiates these relationships, and the resulting trust that staff members have in their manager enables a feeling of security to envelop everyone. Staff members, confident in their roles, are able to raise patient satisfaction and contribute to their organization's bottom line.

Staff meetings are important, and knowing that their opinions are valued, most of the team members attend them. When a staff member contributes a good idea, the manager implements that idea in days, not months. Good managers know the finest ideas come from direct-care staff who notice ways to improve their workplace. Staff members are motivated to keep their ideas flowing because they get satisfaction from seeing their ideas put into practice. They know they will also have a better work environment.

When a manager wants to fill staffing holes, team members cooperate and often volunteer to rearrange their schedules to fill vacancies. They know that when they need time off, their manager will at least put forth a good effort to accommodate them.

THE SMART NURSING PROCESS FOR BUILDING HIGH-PERFORMANCE TEAMS

1. Form relationships.
    Do you want all your nurses to be cookie-cutter nurses, all the same? One secret to building relationships is to encourage

employees to be themselves. It is exhausting to have to keep up a false front. Get to know your nurses' true identities, and show them your own true self. Of course, no one is perfect, but the strengths and weaknesses of individual team members counterbalance each other. The connections between team members can become your greatest strength.

2. Empower your staff.

Nurses need power if you expect them to strive for excellence. A nurse's intuition, honed by many years of education and experience, suggests the right action. Many nurses say intuition is responsible for their most astute decisions. This is how experienced nurses add value to your organization.

Empowered nurses avoid burnout because they control the quality of the care they provide. Psychological principles maintain that people experience reduced stress when they retain control of a situation, even if the situation is negative. And patients are grateful to have such strong advocates working on their behalf.

3. Choose smart strategies.

Your staff members need to understand senior management's perspective in order to work toward organizational success. But many organizations build their strategic plans and then keep them at the board level, far away from the people responsible for making them succeed. That is why they fail. Plans must be living, breathing undertakings. When employees understand your plan, they are able to collaborate and strengthen your whole organization.

Many CEOs sincerely value contributions from all levels of their staff. But some senior managers only value what their managers do. They fail to recognize that it is the employees who make managers successful. Good managers know they can succeed only with plenty of dedicated employees on their team.

4. Remove obstacles.

Take the quiz at the end of this chapter to see where you stand on the teamwork continuum. Ask your team members to identify what they think is holding your team back. Ask outside observers for their opinion. Consult with senior management for their advice. Read books on teamwork and learn from the experiences of others. Network with other facilities to see what works for them.

Prioritize your obstacles and take action to remove them. Don't just continue to analyze.
5. Give feedback.

Feedback is a gift, a personal and professional gift so you can become the best person and have the best team possible. As with any gift, it means more when given with a spirit of generosity and support. Even if the motive is less altruistic, pay attention and evaluate the suggestions objectively. If the feedback seems accurate, incorporate the suggestions into your work.

SUGGESTIONS FOR TEAM LEADERS

1. Delegate decision making.

The best managers enable their nurses to solve patient problems on the spot instead of requiring them to go up and down long chains of command. Delegation promotes patient satisfaction and reduces costs.

Patients become dissatisfied when they are forced to wait while their nurses obtain permission to respond to their needs. Managers who empower their staff members enjoy higher staff competence.

Managers can use the time saved to build the kind of relationships that improve nurse retention. These relationships are the basis for renewed commitment of their staff members.
2. Coach your staff.

Remember the adage, "Give a man a fish and you feed him for a day; teach him *how* to fish and you feed him for a lifetime." Maximize your staff's expertise with coaching.

Coach your staff members to make good decisions instead of telling them what to do. Coaching and granting autonomy complement each other since both access the essence of your employees' greatest strengths.

Coaching creates a path for your employees' ideas to flow. Diverse viewpoints contribute to your success. Managers lose these contributions when staff members are expected to be replicas of one another.
3. Think long term.

Results don't happen overnight. Coaching is an investment that takes time and patience, but corporate results grow quickly when employees are able to contribute their best ideas.

Coaching is a long-term process. Staff members need clear consistent communication and support over a period of time before they understand how to use their best ideas at work.

4. Encourage lifelong learning.

Hire for attitude; train for skills. You leap ahead of health care change when your staff members have lifelong learning habits. Because each employee has different interests, your collective employee intelligence will be comprehensive and an asset to your organization.

Managers can promote lifelong learning by encouraging their employees to have curious minds, to think before acting, and to verbalize their interests and concerns.

5. Be a good role model.

You are more likely to achieve results when you influence your staff by setting an example. If you want to be respected, respect others. If you want your staff to be lifelong learners, be one yourself. The same goes for courtesy, autonomy, and other desired staff attributes.

Productivity and quality gains will reward you.

SUGGESTIONS FOR TEAM MEMBERS

1. Value diversity.

In his book *From Conflict to Creativity*, Sy Landau reveals how to unleash creativity and enhance productivity with or without existing conflict. Health care needs this approach. At times, health care employees spend so much time and energy attacking each other and dealing with the resulting chaos that there is little time left to accomplish any work.

2. Think critically.

Be confident and think for yourself. Good organizations support professionals who use common sense when applying policies and procedures. Professionals are most valuable when they come up with simple cost-effective solutions focused on solving patient problems.

3. Cross-train.

It doesn't make sense to have too many staff on one unit and too few on another. Patient census and acuity change rapidly. Cross-training improves your organization's ability to manage those changes. However, staff members may need to set necessary limits so that others do not exploit their flexibility. Organizations should both train and reward you for broadening your skills.

4. Use synergy.

Synergy occurs when a group achieves more together than the sum of what the group members could have accomplished individually. Some examples of synergy are brainstorming, helping a peer with a difficult admission, and creating an education program for the entire team.

Creating more from less is a good approach while attempting to cope with rising staff shortages and decreasing revenue. Staff members prefer to be productive. The obstacles that hold them back frustrate staff more than anyone.

5. Build your own self-esteem.

Low self-esteem magnifies the imperfections of others. Successful people focus on maximizing their own strengths instead of criticizing those of others. Because the skill mix within the team is complementary, individual weaknesses matter less. And teaching each other is a common team practice that helps individuals become stronger professionals.

Every manager and clinical nurse devises their own way to add high-performance teams to their staffing strategy. Customization is a good way is make sure your high-performance team meets your patients' needs. Many approaches will succeed if you adopt the basic principles of respect, dignity, and creativity.

High-performance teams help you achieve the following:

- manage heavy workloads by allowing nurses to accomplish more with less energy
- experience synergy whereby everyone accomplishes more
- raise the value of your most important asset, intellectual capital, the hearts and minds of your employees
- raise productivity in a cost-effective way
- promote accountability, profitability, and staff retention
- increase the effectiveness of your strategic plan
- view all sides of issues, using peers with diverse perspectives as advisors

- make better decisions with quality input from others, allowing them to actually become smarter
- recognize opportunities within your problems
- encourage staff members to turn conflict into creative solutions

---

QUIZ

Do You Work on a High-Performance Team?

Give yourself 1 point for each YES answer.

Questions for Clinical Staff:

1. Does your work group produce quality care?
2. Is each person accountable for his or her results?
3. Do you feel authentic at work, or are you expected to play a role?
4. Is communication between staff members effective?
5. Is your group productive?
6. Have you eliminated gripe sessions at work?
7. Are you as happy about the success of others as you are about your own success?
8. Do you have fun?
9. Does your group enjoy positive relationships?
10. Do you have positive attitudes?
11. Are you energized by your work?
12. Do staff members innovate and improve your workplace?
13. Are your peers mutually respectful?
14. Do staff members share important information with others instead of hoarding it?
15. Do staff members have an entrepreneurial approach to their job? That is, do they feel as if their organization's success is directly related to the job that they do?

Questions for Managers:

1. When choosing a new staff member, do you consider how she or he will function on your team?
2. Are staff members able to solve employee disputes themselves, or do you have to intervene?
3. Are you a good leader as well as a good manager? ["Leaders do the right things; managers do things right." (Warren Bemis)]
4. Do you discuss staffing goals with your nurses, and then give them autonomy to modify staffing levels as needed?
5. Have you implemented at least 95% of your staff members' suggestions within 30 days?
6. Do you insist on respectful behavior from everyone, no matter what his or her position is?
7. Is your staff productive?
8. Is your nursing turnover less than 5%?
9. Is your rate of medical errors low?
10. Do you focus more effort on long term planning than on managing crises?
11. Is your sense of humor a vital part of your management style?
12. Are your staff meetings well attended?
13. Are you open to diverse opinions from your staff?
14. Are you a good role model?
15. Do you use mandatory overtime for less than five shifts per month?

SCORING:

(For each quiz)

Score:		
	13–15	Give everyone a pat on the back.
	10–12	You are on your way.
	7–9	You have the right idea.
	4–6	Have a talk with your team members.
	0–3	Seek out a great team and ask questions.

PROMOTING TEAMWORK

Our current health care environment needs sensible ways to improve productivity. High-performance teams can help. Try them.

Tips for Clinical Nurses

- Develop your communication skills.
- Use your intuition.
- Manage conflict constructively.
- Be a lifelong learner.
- Learn from your peers.

Tips for Managers

- Be trustworthy.
- Listen to your staff's suggestions.
- Calculate your team's value.
- Explain how staff can help with your strategic plan.
- Be a coach.

Tips for Educators

- Use a team approach from the start.
- Develop a curious mind.
- Have a long-term plan.
- Learn critical thinking.
- Ask experienced nurses for teamwork tips.

CHAPTER 11

Safety:
Preventing Medical Errors

To assume is human.

—Michael S. Smith

Medical errors have hit all-time high. Pick up a newspaper or magazine, watch TV, or talk with a friend, and you will come across messages of concern about patient safety. Browse the web and go to the National Institute of Health Web site (www.nih.gov) to confirm this immense concern.

The Leapfrog Group, composed of a number of Fortune 500 companies, has also expressed grave concerns about patient safety (www.leapfroggroup.org). They have banded together to improve health care by using their collective financial clout, promoting the development of safer practices by recommending specific practices. For example, one practice that they have supported is electronic medical-order entry. This would reduce errors from illegible handwriting and would ensure that new orders are cross-checked against a safety database.

PREVENTING MEDICAL ERRORS

Many causes of medical errors are preventable and within management control. This casts a different light on patient safety, because it makes all health care professionals accountable for our dismal safety record.

The key to improving safety is attitude: the attitude of CEO's and their organizations, and all staff. Having the right safety attitude means that safety is more important than your ego or your convenience.

> *The right safety attitude means that safety is more important than your ego or your convenience.*

COMMON PATIENT INJURIES

What are some causes of common patient injuries?

1. Illegible and vague medical orders that are ripe for misinterpretation
2. Procedures done on the wrong patient
3. Wrong-site surgery
4. Medication errors
5. Emergency room delays
6. Nurses who are powerless to intervene when they report significant patient changes
7. Being reactive instead of proactive, unwillingness to act before a situation becomes a crisis
8. Unwillingness to spend money on prevention
9. Inadequate documentation
10. Lack of communication

Decreasing medical errors is important and urgent. Medical errors cause heartaches for patients, their families, and health care professionals.

The good news is that patient safety is easier to achieve than you might think. My suggestions will focus mainly on nursing solutions that are within your control. Most of the Smart Nursing solutions are free or inexpensive. As you might expect, many of the best ways to improve patient safety is to improve the way that you manage nurses.

Nurses and physicians can collaborate on safety issues. A physician orders a large dose of a medication that has a side effect of lowering blood pressure. The nurse knows that this patient's blood pressure has been in the low/normal range. She reports the patient's blood pressure to the physician and expresses her concern that administering this medication will cause this patient's blood pressure to bottom out. The physician, appreciating the nurse's input, changes the medication order.

SAFETY AND STAFFING

Many of the safest organizations empower their nurses to make staffing decisions. They have the authority to determine the number of staff members needed to provide safe care. These nurses are not given this authority without preparation. Their managers coach them so that they fully understand their unit's staffing strategies. They are also held accountable for their decisions and how well they fulfill their responsibilities. The managers and nurses work as partners to achieve their desired staffing patterns. They trust each other. Nurses working on these units have entrepreneurial attitudes, that is, they feel they have a personal responsibility for their organization's success. A spinoff of cultivating an entrepreneurial attitude is high occupancy.

The following two examples explain the differences between staff who have an entrepreneurial attitude and those who don't.

A 20-bed unit has a census of 19 patients. An outside agency calls asking if the unit has an available male bed. The nurse without an entrepreneurial attitude says, "No. We only have a female bed."

In a similar situation, a nurse with an entrepreneurial attitude says, "Yes, I will take the male admission." She is willing to do the extra work involved in moving the female from the private room into the empty bed, making room for the male admission. Assuming that the transfer and admission are appropriate in other ways, this nurse feels that it is her responsibility to keep the unit full because it will make her organization more successful.

Research (as shown in chapter 2) has indicated that the increase in "failure to rescue" deaths has been due to nurse understaffing. Experienced nurses have been able to point out potential clinical complications early. Now, many of these complications are ad-

dressed too late, when the patient's vital signs have already deteriorated. Fewer patients survive when early symptoms of complications
are missed when there is still time to act.

RISK MANAGEMENT

Nurses as Frontline Risk Managers

Nurses improve the return on your health care investment by decreasing risk. They have the potential to improve patient safety by
functioning as frontline risk managers.

Clinical nurses notice complications early, often in time to prevent
injury. But without management support, nurses cannot act soon
enough to prevent patient injury. Nurses could improve patient
safety and help their organizations avoid expensive litigation if they
had more power and were supported by their CEOs.

For example, a nurse giving medications notices a dropper bottle
in the medication room. She picks it up and reads the label, which
says "hemoccult developer solution." She recalls an article in one
of her nursing journals describing a severe medication error that
occurred when a nurse accidentally put hemoccult developer in a
patient's eyes instead of eyedrops. This error resulted in total blind-
ness for the patient. The nurse knows that the hemoccult developer
didn't belong in the medication room and could be the source of a
potentially serious error. She moves the hemoccult developer to the
utility room. But this near-miss was never investigated. Hospitals
that use near-miss reports to track potential errors decrease actual errors.

CEO Influence on Safety

CEOs are the ones in organizations who set the standard for every
single employee.

From my experience, the safest organizations have *all* had one
common trait, excellent CEOs. Each time, the CEO has been the right
kind of role model. He or she was held in high esteem by the staff,

and there was genuine trust between the staff and their CEO. The CEO's actions have raised staff morale and built commitment.

CEOs in less successful organizations coerce their staff. This promotes distrust and low morale.

Usually the safest organizations are the ones with the best cultures and also the most profitable. One would think that CEOs would want to build a positive culture if for no other reason than to ensure financial success

Many problems within organizations are actually systems problems, problems that nurses are unable to solve independently. Systems problems occur when many departments share the cause, and no one department can solve it on their own. Positive cultures solve systems problems by fostering interdepartmental collaboration. Read the findings by the Harvard study (chapter 2) that describes how nurse powerlessness interferes with patient safety.

SYSTEMS PROBLEMS AND SMART NURSING

Many managers continue to overburden their nurses with increasingly heavy clinical tasks. This requires nurses to work faster and faster instead of allowing them to work smarter.

Managers would raise nurse productivity with Smart Nursing, because tired nurses lose productivity and accuracy. Managers could determine if their issues were systems problems if they listened to nurses. They could then solve the root problems instead of focusing on the symptoms of problems.

Take this example into account: The following responsibilities were the expectations of day shift RNs during their first hour of work: (1) Listen to report. (2) Assess vital signs for all. (3) Prepare pre-op outpatients for surgery. (4) Pour and administer the morning medications. (5) Provide morning physical care. (6) Supervise breakfast.

Because it was impossible to perform that much work in such a short time, the nurses frequently skipped listening to report so that they could finish the rest of their tasks. This placed the organization at risk for serious errors. The following example describes the errors that can occur when nurses don't have enough time to listen to report:

A nurse starts to take vital signs without listening to report. She approaches a patient sitting in a chair outside his room. His name band confirms his identity. The nurse takes his blood pressure un-eventfully. It is only later, after listening to report, that she discovers the patient had a dialysis access catheter inserted in his chest and that he should not have blood pressures taken in one arm. Although taking the blood pressure this time caused no harm, the potential for error was there. Listening to report is necessary for safety even with simple procedures such as vital sign assessment.

The nurse manager correctly recognized this situation as a sys-tems problem. Instead of asking nurses to work harder and faster, she consulted with them and reconfigured some of the tasks: Taking vital signs and performing morning care was reassigned to the night shift LNAs, and outpatient surgeries were assigned to another unit.

The 7-to-3 RNs were then able to perform their work safely and with excellence. Nursing input had enabled the manager to change a flawed system, allowing the nurses to work safer and smarter.

HOW TO IDENTIFY AND SOLVE SYSTEMS PROBLEMS

- Track medical errors, and then identify the root causes. Re-member to take action to eliminate the root causes of problems so that they don't keep recurring.
- Track near-misses. Use near-miss reports to identify high-risk issues. Identify the root causes of the near misses and take action, just as you did for medical errors.
- Maintain a nonpunitive attitude regarding errors. This enables you to obtain necessary data to use in preventing future errors.

We need CEOs, physicians, trustees, and others who recognize nursing value, and support nurses as important health care profes-sionals. Collaboration with nurses will enable organizations to pro-vide the safe and cost-effective care that patients deserve.

Empowerment

Empowering frontline employees enables nurses to become strong patient advocates. Instead of "voices crying in the wilderness," nurses are credible reporters who are taken seriously by both man-agement and physicians. Patient symptoms are acted upon the first time a nurse reports a concern, not after a patient's condition has deteriorated.

Empowered nurses can prevent patient injury caused by unsafe requests from someone with more power. These empowered nurses know that their nurse manager will support their decisions.

An empowered nurse has the authority to prevent inappropriate patient admissions. Patient transfers are often attempted when they do not meet admission criteria. For example, psychiatric patients need medical clearance because mental health units have only a minimal supply of medical equipment. Patients remain safer when they receive care on a properly equipped unit.

Empowering nurses enables you to use a proactive approach. Facilities cut corners at times thinking that they will be lucky. They hope that tragedy in the form of medical errors will not happen to them. But effect follows cause, and serious errors do occur unless you follow precise safety guidelines. If you continually ignore safety protocols, it is only a matter of time before your facility will experience serious medical errors.

- Be proactive. Staff your units safely.
- Be proactive. Investigate near misses.
- Be proactive. Review and scrutinize the habits of physicians and other professionals with patterns of numerous errors.
- Be proactive. Solve root problems before patients are injured.
- Be proactive. Choose safe, long-term solutions over risky quick fixes.
- Be proactive. Manage with integrity instead of spending time and energy on expensive cover-ups.
- Be proactive. Design and test safety protocols for results.
- Be proactive. Listen to your clinical staff.

All of these suggestions are within your control. All of them are free. All of the suggestions would improve patient safety. We have no excuse to ignore them.

EDUCATING ABOUT SAFETY

Our country's high rate of medical errors endangers patients, organizations, and nurses. What everyone doesn't realize is that it is possible to use education to reduce medical errors while still maintaining high productivity standards.

Use the following suggestions to educate yourself. It is important to look at safety in a holistic way, and to demonstrate an intuitive grasp of potentially unsafe situations.

1. Maximize your orientation. Orientation is a time when nurses have an especially high risk of making errors. Take your time. Ask questions, and focus on developing solid safety habits. Orientation is an opportunity to learn as much as you can before being counted as a full-time equivalent. Use it wisely.

2. When it seems that you have to respond to many urgent demands at the same time, take that extra second to clear your mind, relax, and take a deep breath no matter how busy you are. You will find that you will be able to complete your work safely and on time.

3. Use positive self-talk. Say to yourself, "I will work quickly but not so quickly as to make errors. I don't want to rush this treatment and cause heartaches to my patient and myself."

4. Always check medication labels three times!!! Yes! Three times every time!!! Experienced nurses with good safety records find their own errors before giving the medications. For example, after carefully retrieving a medication, during the second check they discover that the medication is wrong. They are then able to replace the medication with the right one.

   Nurses also find that their fast-paced environments can be distracting. Again, they can correct their errors on the second or third check before administering the medication to the patient.

5. Always ask yourself the "5 Rights": **Right** medication; **Right** dose; **Right** time; **Right** route; **Right** patient.

6. Use at least two patient identifiers whenever taking blood samples or administering medications or blood products.

7. Look up unfamiliar medications in reference books.

8. Pay attention to your intuition when something seems wrong.

9. Inquire about questionable situations *before* you administer the medication.

As these safety rules become automatic, you will find that you can work just as fast with them as without them. *Don't ever cut corners on safety practices to save time.*

Using the Smart Nursing strategies is cost-effective and promotes safety with accountability, respect, and empowerment. But any system is only as strong as the staff that carry out the safety protocols. No protocol will ever replace the value of a competent and caring staff who skillfully ensure that the protocols produce the best results possible.

PROMOTING SAFETY

Tips for Clinical Nurses

- Be firm about safety issues
- Clear your mind when you have multiple issues happening at once
- Be holistic about safety issues
- Use positive self-talk to pace yourself
- Listen to patient's concerns about safety

Tips for Managers

- Empower nurses to make safety decisions
- Be proactive
- Build interdisciplinary approaches to safety
- Create a learning organization
- Document near-misses

Tips for Educators

- Develop nurses who have an entrepreneurial attitude
- Encourage your students to have intellectual curiosity
- Explore health care power issues
- Teach nurses to be risk managers
- Encourage students to participate in safety improvement strategies

CHAPTER 12

Diversity: The Magic Is in the Staffing Mix

Empathy makes a leader able to get along well with people of diverse backgrounds or from other cultures.

—Daniel Goleman

People are different. Diversity in the area of health care could be our greatest strength if we embraced diversity instead of rebuking it. Individual variance causes unnecessary conflict when differences are considered as threats. In this chapter, we use the term "diversity" to mean differences of all types—in personality, skills, outlook, and culture.

Some employees prefer looking at the big picture while others thrive by focusing on small details. Certain employees are more people-oriented, while their counterparts would rather concentrate on tasks. Some people relish the limelight, while others find satisfaction working behind the scenes.

Health care management has long rejected diverse viewpoints, considering them as threats to the status quo. Their intentions were often admirable. In their minds, standardization was needed to ensure safety.

However, standardization has failed in all spheres. We have lost the innovation that we needed to remain financially solvent and have not even improved safety, with our medical error rate at an all-time high.

132

Excessive paperwork was generated during the 1980s and 1990s in an attempt to standardize care and improve safety. However, this merely served to consume a lot of time and took nurses away from providing safe care to their patients.

Diversity builds profitability. Organizations have lost valuable market data that could have prevented our current financial problems. When managers cut costs without listening to nurses, they sowed the seed of our current nursing crisis. Nurses haven't volunteered to offer suggestions because they have been censured so many times for having a different perspective. So now, nurses rarely even report many of their concerns.

Organizations must satisfy customer needs if they want to remain competitive. But before satisfying those needs, they must know what those needs are. Organizations need to listen to nurses who are in the best position to listen to patients, and then management will be able to create the kinds of services desired by consumers. Having continual streams of ideas from frontline employees such as nurses ensures financial viability and keeps you ahead of the competition.

Diversity also reduces risk. A balanced mix of personalities decreases risk because everyone looks at various aspects of each problem differently. For example, a seminar participant recounted some workplace conflicts resulting from her manager's habit of focusing on the big picture, while she liked centering on the details. When encouraged to think back to situations when her focus on detail paid off, her face suddenly lit up. "Yes, my organization was sued several years ago, and it was my detailed written notes that provided the necessary documentation needed to win the case." In this instance, both the manager and employee were able to reduce their risk because of their diversity of temperaments.

Respect for diversity forms the foundation for innovation, yet health care has not been very kind to innovators. The powerful status quo usually squashes many novel ideas. You can counteract this tendency by providing a nurturing environment so that innovators can survive. Innovation represents the bridge to our future.

Good managers encourage collaboration between innovators and less inventive employees. Each learns from the other so that both can become more successful.

Diversity is also necessary for teamwork. Teams that represent all personality styles perform better. Their different perspectives help teams overcome obstacles and add value to their organization.

Showcase your diversity. Suppose you have a nurse who excels at categorizing things. With good humor recognize her by saying, "Cindy color-coded all of our keys to save us all a little bit of valuable time." And remember to say thank you. Everyone on your staff needs sincere appreciation.

FIVE WAYS TO CAPITALIZE ON DIVERSITY BY FOCUSING INWARD

1. *Assess your own self-esteem.* Low self-esteem is a lens that distorts the actions of others. Staff with low self-esteem are likely to assess people wrong and undermine them. Some people think if the other person is right than they must be wrong. A struggle about who is right and who is wrong ensues to protect their fragile self-esteem. This kind of competition and sabotage occurs frequently in health care. Skilled nurse managers can end it by making sure that everyone has an equal chance to participate.
2. *Examine your attitude.* People fear change and spend an enormous amount of energy fighting it. Because corporate structures change frequently, ask yourself, "Is this change an innovative way to improve services or is it a threat to basic values such as honesty and commitment to quality?" In the first case, go with the flow, but oppose the change in the second case.
3. *Change yourself first.* We influence others more than we think. An authoritarian approach creates dependency. On the other hand, a staff-friendly culture cultivates the independence necessary for staff to use all of their abilities.
4. *Be flexible.* Good policies create quality and consistency. But policies are black-and-white, while human situations come in shades of gray. Use critical thinking if a policy doesn't make sense. Policies should serve the customer, not the other way around. Organizations should hire professionals to use their judgment and interpret policies on an individual basis.
5. *Have a sense of humor.* Humor decreases stress and improves teamwork. Friendly teasing about differences can actually bond staff members to each other. "That's a good job for you, Sara. I know you'll take care of every detail."

FIVE WAYS TO CAPITALIZE ON DIVERSITY BY FOCUSING OUTWARD

1. *Understand diversity.* We tend to compare ourselves with others. If the other is different, some people automatically think they are wrong. A better approach is to reframe the situation and ask yourself, "What can I learn from this person?"
2. *Show respect.* Respect empowers people because it allows them to be authentic. Staff are more innovative and productive when they can be themselves.
3. *Communicate effectively.* People with different personalities need different approaches. Choose one that will match the other person's expectations. In other words, don't be a one-trick pony. Learn various communication styles so that you can pick the best one for each situation. If you have one or two styles, you may be effective in 25% to 35% of situations. If you have six to eight styles, you have a good chance of being effective in every situation.
4. *Seek areas of agreement.* Search for ways to agree. A list of agreements makes it easier to create enough momentum to overcome points of disagreement. Focusing on the positive can actually make it happen.
5. *Collaborate.* Collaboration is more successful in a diverse environment because of the multitude of ideas from which to choose. When people say, "These results are better than any member of the team could have produced alone," you know that you have achieved success.

I attended my clinical nursing education in New York City at a hospital with a substantial Hispanic population. We learned to speak Spanish, and were taught how to be the right kind of nurse for our patients.

One lesson that I learned was to be flexible. We were asked to listen well, to look at each situation individually, and to remain sensitive to cultural differences.

For example, our Hispanic patients were accustomed to maternity practices that at first seemed foreign to us. But we didn't try to impose our own ideas on them. As we examined their customs, we discovered that most of their customs were just different ways to accomplish the same goals that were in our texts. Occasionally, we made some suggestions to improve the care of their infants. But mostly, we genuinely respected them, built warm relationships, and shared in the joy they experienced with the birth of their children.

Assess how you can use your diversity better. Look inward *and* outward for ways to promote diversity. Welcome people with different personalities and beliefs so that you and your organization can benefit from the magic of the staffing mix.

PROMOTING DIVERSITY

Tips for Clinical Nurses

- Avoid feeling threatened by diversity
- Be flexible
- Understand others
- Seek agreement
- Avoid defensiveness

Tips for Managers

- Question standardized protocols to reduce waste
- Share power
- Be adaptable
- Showcase diversity
- Use diversity to decrease risk

Tips for Educators

- Accept diverse points of views
- Use experiential strategies
- Decrease standardization for students
- Stimulate multiple solutions to challenges
- Encourage students to speak up

CHAPTER 13

Leadership:
Coaching and Mentoring Others

The anger I felt, and continue to feel, about the attacks on the World Trade Center was healthy—the challenge was to put it to work in ways that would make me a stronger better leader.

—Rudolph Giuliani

Mayor Giuliani's comments are especially relevant to health care professionals! Challenges can have positive outcomes with the right approach. The entire health care industry can benefit if nurses use the nursing crisis as an incentive to become strong leaders.

Relationships shape the foundation of leadership, and trust binds this foundation together just as it binds people together. This process builds a sense of community that enables nurses to function at their full professional capacity.

Consider the potential consequences of the lack of trust in the following story:

While waiting in line to place my order at a snack bar, I overheard a conversation between a 9-year-old boy and the snack bar's manager. Apparently the boy's father had given the manager a list of acceptable lunchtime beverages. The boy wanted a root beer, but the manager would not give it to him because it wasn't on his list, thus causing the argument.

137

My thoughts were as follows: A 9-year-old will soon be approached by drug dealers. If this boy can't be trusted to choose a lunchtime beverage, how will he ever be able to make an intelligent decision about whether to use drugs?

I related this story to my daughter's friend, a Gen Xer, and he commented, "Maybe the boy's father plans to give the drug dealer a list of acceptable drugs."

Like the boy's father, health care organizations are failing to trust their nurses and delegate appropriate decision-making authority. This omission has prevented nurses from performing at their full professional capacity.

The best leaders share power and build consensus by coaching and mentoring their employees. They replicate their passion for leadership by encouraging each staff member to seek his or her own individual style. They inspire nurses and other health care professionals to put their hearts and souls into their work. The result of good leadership is the kind of quality care that makes patients whole.

The best leaders delegate decision-making authority to frontline employees such as nurses. One of a leader's most important roles is to help their frontline employees to excel. To achieve this goal, health care managers must delegate enough authority to their nurses so that they can make binding decisions. This act of empowerment allows clinical staff to respond to patient needs at the right time. Delegation also prepares nurses to become future leaders. As nurses operate with greater authority, they will experience professional growth and gain new skills, all of which will provide benefits to their entire organization.

Consider what the Institute of Medicine (IOM) reported after it took a critical look at the working conditions for nurses in America's hospitals:

Enabling nursing staff to collaborate with other health care personnel in identifying high-risk and inefficient work processes and workspaces . . . is also essential . . . Recommendation 6-2. HCOs should provide nursing leadership with resources that enable them to design the nursing work environment and care processes to reduce errors. These efforts must directly involve direct-care nurses throughout all phases of the work design. (IOM, 2004)

Clinical nurses who lead unit projects strengthen their skills in communication, collaboration and negotiation. These skill sets can be used for future projects and can ensure that nurses' voices are heard.

Nurses who are asked to create "variance summaries" each month gain a new understanding about error trends and learn how to improve safety. This important information filters down to the entire staff, enriching the whole unit. Many times, safety suggestions from peers are more easily accepted. Nurses who participate at this level build analytic skills that raise their value to the entire organization. They can use those skills in other venues, making these resources self-renewing. When managers use delegation in this manner, they make large deposits into their organization's intellectual capital fund. Delegation also promotes staff buy-in during times of organizational change because employees are more likely to follow policies that they have created.

When managers delegate wisely, they are able to significantly reduce their own workloads. Do they put their feet up and do nothing? No. They spend their time building relationships with their staff. They also use their time to reflect on how to resolve the root causes of problems instead of being consumed by responding only to the symptoms of the problem. Managers who delegate effectively find that staffing issues take less time because high nursing satisfaction promotes collaboration. Empowered clinical nurses have higher job satisfaction because they can solve their own problems without going up and down a long chain of command.

COACHING AND MENTORING

Mentors and coaches are valuable tools to use in solving two pressing health care issues: patient safety and staff retention. Apply your organization's goal when choosing mentors. Mentoring can be formal or informal as when a mentor remains alert for spontaneous opportunities during the course of daily work.

As managers, you are ever alert to employee turnover. According to a 2002 employee turnover study by the American Healthcare Association, the national turnover rates for long-term care are 48.9% annually (www.AHCA.org, 2003). Many acute care facilities have high nursing turnover rates as well.

5 Ways to Use Coaching and Mentoring to Retain Employees

1. Use "stay interviews." Some companies enjoy high retention because they take time to talk with employees about remaining onboard. One employee who experienced a stay interview described it this way: "It makes a difference to have something other than your standard review. And, I feel appreciated when my manager takes the extra time."

2. Ask yourself the following question: Are my employees receiving a good return on their investment of time, talent and money? When 25 global talent leaders got together for a think tank, key issues regarding employee engagement and retention were discussed. One of their key findings was that employees need to feel that they have a return on their investment in the company (Kaye, 2003).

3. Give your nurses enough support. Many nurses think of safer ways to perform their job but won't contribute those ideas without support. Mentors are in a good position to promote staff safety initiatives.

4. Spot employee dissatisfaction early. Mentors are in an ideal position to monitor employee satisfaction. They notice the beginning of staff cynicism early. When mentors are unable to intervene, they will know how to find someone else who can respond to the situation.

5. Be a good role model. CEOs and nursing directors should be the finest mentoring models. Employees respond well to seeing clear corporate values in action and having a model of excellence to live up to.

One excellent nurse leader was in the process of handling a common clinical situation that led to a discussion to better understand the details of the situation. I made the following observations: The leader avoided a confrontational approach and kept an open mind to accurately absorb the details of the situation. But she did not gloss over potential sources of conflict. Instead, she used systematic open- and close-ended questions to obtain an abundance of accurate information. Her attitude also prevented staff defensiveness, and facilitated employee growth. This leader later shared her thoughts with me.

I am always one who wants the truth and respects the truth from my staff. We can learn more about what happened besides what was reported to us. Sometimes these things take on a life of their own. I am a firm believer that everyone should learn problem solving and decision-making skills. My job is so much more than being a manager. It is being a leader and a role model.

Staff who work in this type of environment can perform at their full professional capacity.

INVOLVE NURSES IN STRATEGIC PLANNING

Most health care organizations use strategic plans to guide the decisions they make. Strategic plans tend to focus on understanding external influences and examine whether their organization has achieved a good fit with their environment. Common external challenges studied by strategic planners are the supply and demand of employees and third-party reimbursement trends. Strategic plans also examine internal strengths such as the presence of intellectual capital (such as experienced nurses). Of course strategic plans are more complex, but these are especially relevant to nurses.

The present low supply of nurses (an external industry challenge) interferes with an organization's ability to offer all the services that patients need. Many organizations would expand if they could hire enough nurses.

Organizations that minimize nursing value think a nurse is a nurse is a nurse. But that is not so. Cross-trained nurses, specialty nurses, or those with strong leadership abilities are value-added employees.

The point here is not to compare different nurses, but to illustrate that all nurses should seek to add value to their organizations. Another important point is that facilities would benefit if they stopped undervaluing their nurses and started including them as important players in their strategic plans. In terms of chess, nurses should not be viewed as pawns, but as more powerful players in the health care game.

Strategic plans become more meaningful when you involve clinical nurses who are crucial to your success. Consider using the following techniques to involve nurses in strategic planning:

1. Hold focus groups composed of nurses to elucidate valuable nursing perspectives.

2. Ask for positive and negative feedback regarding your organizational culture and how it affects nurse productivity.
3. Review your corporate values. Do you practice these values consistently? Are they compatible with staff values?
4. Invite your clinical nurses to share their ideas on nurse recruitment and retention and other important issues.
5. Discuss the benefits for all staff members when nurses share their skills with each other.
6. Ask yourself, Do I identify my nurses' skills in my strategic plan? You should know what skills your nurses have. (See the skill assessment sheet in the appendix for chapter 17.)

- Which nurses are cross-trained?
- What nonclinical skills, computer literacy, artistic ability, or public speaking, are available to you?
- How can you best support information sharing? Reward nurses who are willing to utilize a large number of their skills. When nurses are generous with their abilities, managers should be generous in return.
- Align nursing with other departments.
- Successful organizations know how to induce their departments to work together. They use synergy to raise productivity. This means that no department is more important than another, and they avoid turf wars.
- What attracts and retains exceptional talent?
- The best nurses want to work with competent peers who are similarly interested in excellence. Many times, these exceptional nurses will recruit others just like them because they value working in such positive environments.
- Expand your employees' capabilities.
- What are the effective rewards for lifelong learners? If you are a clinical nurse, become a lifelong learner so that you have more to offer your employer.
- Cultivate new leaders. Teach the components of leadership—communication, respect, and vision. Let your staff practice on small projects, and give them feedback.

Leadership excellence results in the following benefits:

- high nurse retention
- decreased medical errors

- high nurse satisfaction.
- high staff skill base
- a positive culture
- a sense of community
- high return on investment on nurses
- positive public relations messages

Delegation ideas:

- Invite nurses to be on-unit educators.
- Encourage them to take responsibility for QA projects.
- Ask nurses to present patient-education programs.
- Provide opportunities for nurses to participate in shared governance.
- Involve nurses in joint projects with other health care organizations.

Quality increases when you involve nurses in unit leadership. Delegation reduces nurse turnover because the staff feels valued. Practicing the Smart Nursing strategies of respect, simplicity, flexibility, integrity, communication, and professional culture will help you build a strong foundation as you build your leadership skills.

SUCCESSFUL COACHING IN ACTION

Linda Pullins, VP
Marion General Hospital (Ohio)

At Marion General Hospital, in Marion, Ohio, great changes are evident, as the result of 2 years of intense work with the nursing staff. Morale was at an all-time low, there were unfilled nurse manager positions, near-misses were rising, and agency staffing costs were through the roof, with so many unfilled RN positions.

Linda Pullins, VP of Patient Care Services, planned a bold move that would move some of her best nurses out of bedside staffing and other positions into the role of professional coaches, in an effort to get to the root problem of what was going on in patient care. Nurses were invited to participate in a 1-year initiative that would place them directly at the bedside, working with RNs to improve their care management and critical-thinking skills. All were guaranteed that they could transfer back into their original positions at the end of one year.

A proposal was shared with the CEO and Medical Staff Executive Committee that would entail hiring additional agency nurse staffing to cover some of the positions. Outcomes and success measures were identified along with metrics to measure along the way. The idea of pulling good nurses away from taking care of patients was met with resistance and disdain at various levels. The idea of bringing in some select consultant interventions also was met with skepticism. Why couldn't we just fix this ourselves?

Linda knew that this was not going to be a quick fix, for patient care had not gotten to this level overnight and she needed to be clear on what the priorities for the coaches would be. The professional coaches spent 3 weeks in didactic and classroom discussions, learning about emotional intelligence, how coaching was different from precepting, how we would address the numerous problems that they would encounter, and how the staff would accept them.

Within 6 months the start of a turnaround was apparent, as the coaches would share their own stories and examples of how far both they and the staff had come. This was certainly not an easy journey, nor was every week filled with successes. Many tears were shed, along with many good laughs, but the joy of taking care of patients was coming back to Marion General!

Marion General now enjoys the following: Press Ganey Patient Satisfaction has moved from the 4th percentile to the 86th percentile on the inpatient survey. Retention is now at 94%, Employer of Choice scores from the employees is at a 5-year-high, and 56 RNs were successfully recruited in 1 year—three times the normal recruitment! Our patients, staff, physicians, and new employees tell us that there is something different about Marion General.

It can happen, but it must happen at the bedside, working side by side to deal with the stressful and complicated care issues of today. We are a better organization, and we are taking better care of our patients with this work. As Arthur Ashe once said, "To achieve greatness, start where you are. Use what you have. Do what you can."

PROMOTING LEADERSHIP

Tips for Clinical Nurses

- Build leadership skills
- View leadership as a challenge
- Follow up on your initiatives
- Seek accountability
- Be generous with praise and support

Tips for Managers

- Use relationships to connect with your staff
- Build consensus
- Create a shared vision
- Value your intellectual capital
- Use nurses to increase your organization's success

Tips for Educators

- Be a leadership role model
- Maintain frequent contact with nurse leaders
- Give students feedback on their leadership work
- Encourage students to follow current health care leadership issues
- Encourage students to build a vision for the future

CHAPTER 14

Problem-Solving Strategies: Creating Opportunities From Challenges

Your world will be different, and I can't teach you how to solve the problems you will encounter. But I can teach you how to think. If you know how to think, you can solve any problem that comes your way.

—Fritz Bendel, 1955 (author's father)

Within every problem lie the seeds of opportunity. Sowing seeds of opportunity is important, but the course of this kind of change is not always even. New ideas often follow failure and need time to take root and grow. Our many health care challenges constitute important opportunities for all health care professionals.

We need nurses who are able to generate solutions to our challenges. Clinical staff members are well positioned to develop solutions because they see the problems firsthand. Health care executives without clinical experiences need the perspectives of clinical staff if they want to be effective leaders.

This chapter describes the process of transforming problems into opportunities by examining basic problem-solving strategies and suggesting how those strategies can be applied to health care. These strategies involve two main categories: managing thoughts and managing people. Most specific suggestions have elements of both.

Using your thoughts to solve basic problems involves analysis and synthesis. *Analysis* occurs when you break a whole down from a complex to simpler form. *Synthesis* is the reverse, a process of taking the elements from a product and combining them to form the same outcome or recombining them to form another complex outcome.

Think about the following simple analogy of analysis using ordinary saline. When you partially break saline down into its elements, you get sodium and water. To completely break it down into its most elemental form, you must also break the water down into hydrogen and oxygen and the salt into sodium and chlorine.

One health care example of using analysis is the examination of relationships.

Relationships are a complex process involving trust, respect, and other components. Each of those components can be broken down further. For example, respect can be broken down into self-love, open-mindedness, and other qualities.

Synthesis is the process of recombining the basic elements. In the case of saline, you can recombine the salt and water to get saline again; or you can recombine them differently to get stronger saline or a less concentrated version; or you can add other substances such as sugar and get dextrose with saline.

In the case of relationships, trust and respect can be combined to form relationships; or you can add improved communication techniques to form stronger and better relationships. Relationships themselves are a component of other complex issues such as nurse retention, negotiation, and networking.

Many of the concepts in Smart Nursing are the result of breaking issues down into simpler forms and then exchanging the ideas between different disciplines such as education and business.

The use of bar codes to improve safety is another example of a practice from another discipline being successfully adopted by health care.

A book describing the unity of knowledge on a larger scale is *Consilience: The Unity of Knowledge* by Pulitzer Prize–winning author Edward O. Wilson. Wilson shows that natural science, social science, and mathematics have common components.

The purchase of an ordinary Megabucks lottery ticket is an example of consilience. When you decide to buy a ticket, you use both mathematics and psychology. Your choice involves assessing the probability of winning (mathematics), and assessing your attitude toward risk (psychology). For example, are you a risk taker or a risk-averse person?

Many of the ideas in Smart Nursing have evolved from exchanging ideas between various disciplines. The following examples outline the similarities of nursing and marketing.

- Nurses have credibility with customers.
- Marketing requires credibility with customers.
- Nursing involves effective connections with customers.
- Marketing requires effective connections with customers.
- Nurses are experts at assessing patient needs.
- Marketing requires expert knowledge about customer needs.

HEALTH CARE CHALLENGES

You can use this process to transform health care challenges into opportunities by creating your own innovations. Review some of the following health care challenges: safety, role change, productivity, and innovation. These challenges are the source of many nursing opportunities.

Safety

Nurses are risk managers. They notice potential problems early and build positive patient relationships.

Solving problems early allows organizations to decrease their risk, because early nursing interventions prevent patient injury. In the event an error does occur, patients who have developed good relationships with staff are less likely to sue. Patients often start litigation because they feel that "no one cared."

Organizations have caused many of their own safety problems by using heavy-handed tactics to increase nurse productivity. One of these tactics is the "speed-up." Speed-ups require nurses to work faster and faster without regard for consequences. Speed-ups have become an obstacle to patient safety, because they have caused nurse fatigue and prevented nurses from assessing patients often enough. Smart Nursing strategies remove this kind of obstacle to productivity and allow nurses to work smarter instead of just faster. This is one reason why Smart Nursing strategies are more important than ever.

- Quantify the role of nursing as frontline risk managers. A nurse who prevents litigation may save the organization over $500,000.
- Empower nurses to make safety decisions at the patient level.
- Provide safe staffing levels.

If you are a nurse manager or charge nurse, you too have many opportunities to improve safety.

- Express your perspective to senior management.
- Support your nurses, prevent burnout, and show your organization how you can increase productivity with autonomous nurses.

Role Change

Times are changing. In the future, nursing roles will become more advisory and less regulatory. The Internet has enabled patients to collect abundant data, but this does not help them to acquire skills needed to interpret this proliferation of information. Patients will need professional advice to enable them to make smart health care decisions. Nurses are ideally positioned to be advisors to patients, and also well positioned to advise their own leaders.

Nurses are best positioned to fill this emerging advisory role.

To fulfill these roles, nurses will need to expand their outlook. They need to envision management's big picture, as well as their own perspectives, and to think about the larger context affecting these issues. Many times, nurses with legitimate requests limit their success by viewing issues only from their own individual perspective.

Nurses know that patient care success depends on framing their explanations in terms of the patient's point of view. The same is true with management.

Nursing is an important part of your organization's investment in human resources. In the past, facilities have unreasonably slashed nursing budgets. Cost cutting may be necessary, but nurses can best advise their organizations about where to make the cuts without reducing the quality of care. Nurses may advise management to forego expensive building or redecoration in favor of scheduling an adequate number of clinical staff. Listen to them. Act on their reasoned recommendations

Nursing, the most respected of all professions, builds patient trust. Nurses notice patient needs because they spend the most time listening to patients. At present, we are losing this important patient information. Organizations need to capture this data because it is valuable market research. Nurses who advise their organizations are able to identify new services that are needed by patients. For example, nurses and social workers first identified the need for subacute units.

When patients complain about gaps in medical services, explore those complaints. Consider them as important market research. Then, reframe those complaints into opportunities.

Suppose that the patients complain about a lack of transportation. Bring those complaints to management, and reframe them into opportunities. For instance, this may be a good opportunity to start a new shuttle service or to add stops to an existing one.

Frame your requests in terms of benefits to your organization, and show that your requests bring value. For example, "My request will attract new patients." "Although this idea will cost $1,000 to implement, it will decrease expenses by $2,200 annually." "If you change from X to Y, you will double the return on your investment."

Productivity

Productivity is one of our most important issues. Management has tried to raise productivity the wrong way—by insisting that nurses care for too many patients. This practice has caused a rapid rise in our medical error rate, and decreased nurse productivity, because overworked nurse complete less work, not more.

However, the pressure for high nurse productivity will continue because of escalating medical costs. What we need is more collaboration between nurses and managers to find ways to improve nurse productivity without raising the medical error rate. Nurses, as frontline employees, notice ways to streamline their practice in their day to day work.

Sometimes these potential improvement seem too small to bother with, and the nursing staff disregards them. But these potential improvements are very important. For instance, when nurses share small improvements, the discussion often stimulates other nurses to add their ideas. Before you know it, they come up with a faster way to work.

Suppose you find a way to save 10 minutes. When you multiply the 10 minutes by only 100 nurses and then by 365 days, you end up with over 6,000 hours saved per year. From my experience, the best organizations have employees who create continuous streams of small innovations.

If more nurses adopted this philosophy, and were supported by their employers, patients would be able to receive safe care without as much cost.

Innovation

Every nurse can innovate. Assess your own strengths and weaknesses, and then choose to participate in the opportunities that spark your interest.

People gravitate toward certain areas, melding their experiences with their own interests. Be open to new experiences. Be willing to accept opportunities by turning weaknesses into strengths.

In 1995, health care problems resulted in my own reconsideration of nursing as a career. But I reframed the problem into an opportunity. I thought, "Health care problems could be an opportunity for nurses who were willing to work toward positive change." I knew that in order to be successful, I would need better skills of influence.

If you feel limited regarding skills of influence, master them. These are learnable skills. I learned public speaking by joining Toastmasters. You can too. I learned to write for publication by joining a local writers group. You can do the same. Use the nursing shortage as motivation to learn new skills, and to change your work environment.

> *Health care problems are an opportunity for nurses who are willing to work toward positive change.*

Ask yourself what issues are most important.

- Do you want to focus on building a more respectful workplace?
- Do you want to lobby for more autonomy?
- Do you want to participate in marketing?

Identify the skills that you will need to learn. Make a plan, take action, and then go ahead and learn them.

No time? I learned these skills while I was working 44 hours a week as a nurse, taking call 1 day a week, driving two teenage children to all of their activities, and going to graduate school one night a week for 5 years.

I devised the "hour-a-day plan," spending 1 hour a day on my project 6 days a week. I did my homework when my daughters were doing theirs. Try it. You will be amazed at what you will be able to accomplish.

If you are willing to accept these opportunities, you might need to examine the way that you learn. Knowing their own learning style helps people to become more successful students.

Focus on the following actions to maximize your personal and professional growth:

- Nurture your natural curiosity.
- Become a lifelong learner.
- Be persistent.

Nurture Your Natural Curiosity

We all were naturally curious as children. As we mature, we tend to lose this childlike curiosity to different degrees. Nurturing your natural curiosity reconnects you with your creativity and provides you with new opportunities. Your patient safety record will probably improve when you exercise your natural curiosity because it prompts you to follow up on your hunches. Have you ever noticed something odd about a patient? Has natural curiosity led you to check out those symptoms? Haven't you averted medical errors when your curiosity compelled you to check things out?

Using your natural curiosity also keeps you young at heart. A curious mind rejuvenates people, keeps them young, and promotes healthy living.

One way to start restoring your professional curiosity is by brainstorming, which can be done individually as well as in groups. How?

- Choose a topic that interests you.
- Choose a day when you have a few hours of free time.
- Find a quiet spot.
- Clear your mind, and open it to new ideas.
- Write down all of your ideas without judging them—you can weed out the impractical ones later.

Suppose that you witness an incident of disrespect and want to take action. Start brainstorming and see how many action ideas you can generate. I came up with the following 13 ideas in just 3 minutes. You could probably generate many more ideas if you take more time. Write down every idea first.

Sample actions to respond to disrespectful behavior:

1. Build staff self-esteem.
2. Use humor.
3. Be assertive.
4. Talk with the offender privately.
5. Talk with the nurse manger.
6. Talk with senior management.
7. Ask senior management to come to the unit and witness the offensive behavior.
8. Write an article about respect in your newsletter.
9. Recommend that the education department offer classes on anger management.
10. Work with other departments, and take group action.
11. Address this issue at your professional association.
12. Collaborate with physicians.
13. File a complaint with the offender's licensure board.

Now, give brainstorming a try by yourself. Clear your mind, then take 5 or 10 minutes to brainstorm about one of the following topics, or choose another topic:

- Increasing nurse productivity
- Working with management as partners
- Using nurses as risk managers
- Recognizing nurses as marketers

Take out a sheet of paper and number it 1 to 25. Write your topic on the top and start brainstorming, writing all of your ideas down.

Afterwards, prioritize your ideas by numbering them one through 25 according to how much they interest you. Then review the top five and consider how much each topic is needed by your organization or the health care industry. Then choose one or two ideas to pursue further and to take action.

Become a Lifelong Learner

Nurses need to keep learning throughout their lives. Articles in every industry worldwide recommend that employees be lifelong learners. It is the best way to manage change and to remain employable. Nurses who have failed to expand their skills have contributed to the nursing crisis. Health care is a rapidly changing industry. Nurses need to keep up clinically, but they also need to become just as proficient with skills of influence such as *communication*, *negotiation*, and *persuasion*.

Be willing to step outside your comfort zone. Too often, people feel reluctant to try new skills because they enjoy a feeling of security within familiar environments. So they wait to change until they have to. They consider their comfort zones as secure sanctuaries and limit their chances for success. Learning new skills provides intellectual stimulation. People need intellectual stimulation to thrive not just survive. As a result, lifelong learners tend to be among the happy people because they continue their journey of personal and professional growth throughout their lives.

Be Persistent

When you learn a new skill, it is easy to get discouraged. Everyone experiences doubts when others exceed their skill level. It is all right to take "baby steps." The secrets to succeeding with learning new information are to be persistent, use positive self-talk, and reward yourself every now and then.

The process of learning something new can be slow in the beginning until you reach a critical mass. (You must put forth a large effort for a small reward; after you reach the critical mass, you will achieve larger rewards with smaller efforts.) Eventually, you will have learned enough to start feeling competent. You will need more practice to achieve excellence, but you are on your way at that point.

Use positive self-talk along the way such as, "Of course I still make some mistakes, I am a beginner at this." "No one was born with this skill. Everyone was a beginner at one time just like me." "Eventually, I will be an expert in this skill."

Give yourself a reward after you have succeeded with one of your baby steps. Take an afternoon off, get a manicure, and plan lunch with a friend. Rewards help you to enjoy the process and celebrate each level of your success.

Remember, opportunity knocks, and it is knocking loudly on nursing's door. But nothing will happen until you take action. You must open the door to opportunity if you would like to enjoy this kind of success.

TURNING PROBLEMS INTO OPPORTUNITIES

Tips for Clinical Nurses

- Be creative
- Rethink common practices
- Look for an easy way without sacrificing safety or quality
- Read widely
- Question the status quo

(continued)

Tips for Managers

- Use group brainstorming
- Maintain strong connections with senior management and communicate nursing input
- Increase the return on your human resource investment
- Support staff problem-solving
- Encourage group projects to take advantage of synergy

Tips for Educators

- Teach analysis and synthesis of issues
- Look for input from other industries
- Value multiple solutions to problems
- Focus on future needs
- Prioritize health care challenges

Part IV

Looking to the Future

CHAPTER 15

Benefits to Groups Outside Nursing: How CEOs, Physicians, Trustees, and Managed Care Professionals Can Help

---

Seek first to understand, then to be understood.

—Stephen R. Covey

WHY NON-NURSES SHOULD BE INTERESTED IN SMART NURSING

Health care needs many perspectives to solve the nursing crisis. Consumers, physicians, CEOs, and trustees are more effective if they have a good understanding of nursing issues. This understanding promotes better management and more effective interactions with nurses.

The stakes are high: Health care costs are increasing, and the medical error rate has escalated. Many nurses have left health care, and physicians are also being squeezed by the system. CEOs and trustees have the frustrating task of retaining their nursing staffs while at the same time trying to balance their budgets. These problems are especially difficult in health care's current environment of financial cutbacks.

Health care companies administer Medicare and Medicaid programs with mixed reviews. More government involvement in man-

159

aged health care is a strong possibility. Whether this trend continues depends on how well facilities resolve their present challenges. Without better outcomes, Americans may prefer to have a single, non-profit agency administer health care. Private managed-care organizations may find reduced demand for their services and may have to fight for survival.

Consider some of Smart Nursing's benefits to various non-nurse groups:

Benefits to Consumers

- Patients receive safer care with high RN-to-patient ratios. Research, described in the introduction, confirms that even one additional patient added to an RN's assignment substantially raises the complication rate for both medical and surgical patients.
- Satisfaction levels climb when patients receive timely nursing interventions.
- Education provided by nurses promotes wellness.
- Simplified procedures are easy for patients to understand.
- Flexibility enables patients to receive care that is designed for their individual needs.

Benefits to Physicians

- Physicians improve their own quality of care when alert nurses report potential complications that enable physicians to intervene quickly.
- Nursing perspectives added to medical viewpoints promote comprehensive patient care.
- Nurse-physician partnerships save time as when nurses quickly summarize patient events for physicians.
- With enough nurses, physicians can expand their medical practices to meet patient need.
- Physician delegation to nurses reduces medical cost.

Benefits to CEOs and Trustees

- Nurses are the most trusted professionals within your organization. They build positive relationships with your customers and function as your ambassadors.

- Nurses are your organization's frontline risk managers. They notice potential problems early enough to prevent injury. Listen to them.
- Excellent patient care and high patient satisfaction attracts new patients.
- High staff satisfaction reduces human resource outlays.
- Nurses are valuable market researchers. Patient requests often indicate the need for new services.

Benefits to Managed Care Professionals

- An intelligent mix of physicians and nurses results in the most cost-effective care.
- Empowering nurses to make decisions at the patient level reduces bureaucracy.
- Nurse case managers promote a variety of patient choices.
- Excellent customer service by nurses raises managed care profitability.
- Nurses build positive relationships with your providers.

USING SMART NURSING TO ACHIEVE THESE BENEFITS

Smart Nursing strategies potentially can improve the work environment in all types of health care organizations. They provide a solid foundation to develop a culture based on positive and respectful relationships.

Accountability is a form of respect. When you hold nurses accountable for results *and* delegate enough decision-making authority, they can do their best work.

In fact, some facilities are capitalizing on using nursing knowledge and the consistency of nursing's presence by using them as advisors to physicians.

An article in *Modern Healthcare* (Morrissey, 2002) describes how some medical facilities are using nurse specialists to coach doctors regarding effective medical protocol:

It's not unusual for a nurse to approach a physician at Hackensack [NJ] University Medical Center and talk about the right clinical steps to take on behalf of a patient. Surprisingly, it's not unusual for the doctor to take direction from the nurse. But it's for an unusually good reason. The impact of this collegial exchange, and the program that encourages it, is so evident at the 635-bed hospital that the practice of using clinically specialized nurses to monitor and prompt doctors is becoming routine in cardiac and pulmonary care, where the approach was first tried during the past few years . . . The benefits for hospital operations include dramatically higher compliance with proven standards of clinical treatment, along with business bonuses that include lower cost per case and the opportunity to earn millions in extra revenue by improving outcomes and freeing up beds faster. (p. 36)

So why do some doctors continue to treat nurses with disrespect? According to another *Modern Healthcare* (Tieman, 2002) article more than 30% of nurses knew a nurse who had quit because of poor treatment by a physician. This information is based on a study by the Voluntary Hospital of America (VHA).

Ronstein said 92% of respondents said they had witnessed disruptive physician behavior such as inappropriate conflict involving verbal or even physical abuse of nurses. All of the respondents identified a direct link between such behavior and nurse recruitment and retention challenges. Yelling and "condescending behavior" constituted the vast majority of the abuse doctors inflict on their nurse colleagues. (Tieman, 2002, p. 26)

Physicians have traditionally used interactions with nurses as a way to vent their stress. This is no more right than parents who try to relieve stress by abusing their children. Anyone victimizing another person is wrong. Physicians need to find more mature stress relief measures.

This treatment of nurses decreases physician success. Suppose a patient overhears her doctor speaking rudely to an office nurse. Don't you think that the patient lowers her opinion of that doctor? Disrespectful behavior interferes with patient-physician relationships, and may even lead to litigation.

Physician liability costs have escalated. Respectful treatment of others may reduce this liability. Nurses reduce physician liability because they frequently notify physicians about complications before their patients experience permanent disability or die. You could hire an extra nurse and pay his or her salary for 100 years before you reach $5 million, a common award in medical liability suits (calculated by using $50,000 as the nurse's salary).

Another reason for nurses and physicians to treat each other with respect is because they share a common problem. Both have lost control of their practices resulting in a new professional dilemma:

not enough time to provide adequate patient care. Several physicians have asked me to include some ideas for them in this book because many physicians have become just as disenchanted with the health care system as nurses have. Perhaps physician dissatisfaction is one cause for their negative treatment of nurses.

How Physicians Can Raise Their Own Satisfaction

1. Work as partners with other health care staff.
2. Combine your strength to push for positive change.
3. Reduce your liability by listening to other health care professionals.
4. Empower and support nurses. This enables you to reduce some of your own responsibilities.
5. Support advanced practice nurses (legislation increasing their autonomy). Advance practice nurses add to your own success.
6. Working cooperatively with nurses is energy enhancing; conflict is energy draining.
7. Achieve superior patient care outcomes using synergy, achieving better work in a group than working individually.

How Physicians Can Raise Nurse Satisfaction

1. Genuinely respect nurses as important professionals. More than 75% of communication is nonverbal. Unless you feel genuine respect, your body language will display your true feelings.
2. Educate yourself about nursing. Physicians often aren't aware of what nurses are capable of and what nurses legally can and cannot do. Familiarize yourself with your state's nurse-practice act so that you know what nurses are legally allowed to do. Many physicians take nurses for granted and don't value their work.
3. Appreciate nurses. Nurses are an extra pair of eyes and ears for physicians. Observant nurses warn physicians about impending patient complications in time to prevent death or permanent disability. Show appreciation by using nurse assessments. Give appropriate praise for nurses who do their jobs well.

4. Communicate with courtesy. Nurses need respectful communication to achieve excellent performance. It's time to break the old habits of superiority. It's time to consider nurses as equals.
5. Use nursing data. Patient care suffers when nursing input is ignored. We can no longer continue to make errors caused by reluctance to consider all of the patient data.

Consider the following example of a physician using nursing data to improve patient care: A nurse notices that a psychiatric patient appears anxious. He reviews her medications and notices that she has medication available to relieve her anxiety. However, he also notices that the dosage, although not harmful, would probably cause this patient to sleep much of the day, interfering with her ability to attend therapy groups. He contacts the physician and requests a lower dosage of the medication so that his patient can relieve her anxiety but also attend groups.

As health care workplaces become more respectful, patients will enjoy improved care. My hope is that patients and caregivers will find new ways to work together.

SMART NURSING STRATEGIES FOR NON-NURSES

Patient Safety

Despite the negatives, there are many ways that CEOs, trustees, and physicians can improve health care. Our health care system has many positive features. We have the most comprehensive health care data bank in the world, and the freedom we enjoy has the potential to leverage that knowledge into superior results. Health care staff members are both knowledgeable and compassionate.

Non-nurses can use Smart Nursing strategies to maximize these assets. Respect, flexibility, simplicity, culture, integrity, and communication are all good tools for non-nurses. An added advantage is that these strategies are free of charge.

What some non-nurses have found difficult is eliminating some of health care's sacred cows. We must abandon our rigid hierarchical system that places physicians and managers high above frontline employees such as nurses. We must utilize all of the best information, whether the source of that information is a physician, a nurse, or a manager. And we must learn to communicate with each other with courtesy, and respect.

Daniel Goleman (2002) shares the following example of how CEO and physician attitudes can increase medical errors:

> They don't have enough real contact with people in their organizations. . . . These leaders are clueless, or in denial about the reality of their organization. While they may believe that everything is fine, they have in fact created a culture in which no one dares to tell them anything that might provoke them, especially bad news. That kind of silence can come at a very high price.
>
> One physician . . . told us: "In the culture of hospitals, a nurse who corrects a doctor—telling him he wrote too many zeroes in an order for patient's meds—can get her head bitten off. If medicine were to adopt the zero tolerance for mistakes that sets the norm for the airline mechanic industry, we'd cut medical errors drastically." (p. 193)

Nurses have complained all through the 1990s that short staffing is unsafe. And they were absolutely right. The large research studies described in the introduction have determined that even one patient added to a nurse's assignment greatly increases the medical error rate.

Bureaucracy

Whatever health care system is used by patients, bureaucracy has consumed far too many of our scarce health care resources.

- Indirect care (i.e., maintaining records, documentation) has become so time-consuming that direct care time at the bedside has become more limited.
- Nurses have little time to listen to patients and give emotional support. In many circumstances, emotional support may be even more important than physical care.
- Without proper direction, patients omit necessary follow-up of treatments or medications.

Our fast-paced health care environment requires quick responses. Nurses would be able to decrease some of our medical errors if they were allowed to take quick actions to prevent injury. Consider the following perspective about power, and how Alan Weiss (2000) views the relationship between powerlessness and bureaucracy:

> There is a grand myth extant in organizational life that "power corrupts," a vestige of an overzealous reading of Edmund Burke 200 years ago. Actually, the opposite position is true in business: *powerlessness corrupts.*
>
> When employees are truly powerless—that is, they cannot make decisions which influence the outcome of their work—they will create artificial power.
>
> Psychologically, most people can't remain healthy if they are engaged in a job, which they routinely cannot influence. This is a sometimes desperate and always encumbering attempt to control their environment and bring some influence to their work lives.
>
> What we encounter as customers are ridiculous policies, rude comments, harsh treatment and deliberate sabotage. That's because employees who feel powerless create artificial power, which we generally refer to as "bureaucracy." (Excerpted with permission from "Leadership for a New Millennium," by Alan Weiss, Ph.D., copyright (2000) Alan Weiss, all rights reserved. Full article available on his Web site http://www.summit-consulting.com.)

Non-nurses achieve more success when they examine the following three aspects of their organizations: structure, process, outcomes.

Structure

Analyze your formal and informal power structure. Ask yourself, Who actually has the power? Think about whether a simplified structure would improve outcomes. Would you benefit by building in more flexibility so that you can respond to rapid industry changes? Does your structure help or hinder your customers' well-being? What about your corporate values? Are they a practical guide or merely abstractions?

Process

Do you suffer from bureaucratic gridlock? Would sensible downsizing allow you to function better? Consider whether simplifying procedures would streamline your processes without decreasing quality. How could employee autonomy help? Are you satisfied with your employee performance? What kinds of controls do you have in place?

What are your strategies to stimulate innovation by frontline employees? Do your employees exhibit critical thinking skills?

Outcomes

What is your safety record? What scores have you achieved in patient satisfaction surveys? Are you profitable? Is your profitability consistent? If not, why not? Do you produce a quality product or service? Are your employees satisfied? What is your employee turnover rate? Would your employees recommend your organization to others? Overall, would you describe your outcomes as progress or regress?

Look inward. Look at your structures, processes, and outcomes. Then use the Smart Nursing principles to make improvements.

Patient Satisfaction

Patient satisfaction is related to profitability because a good reputation is what attracts patients.

Many times, people meeting nurses give feedback about their medical issues. For example, consider the following experience a fellow professional shared with me during a conference: He was fighting depression and went to his primary physician, who responded by prescribing an antidepressant. "It's quicker to write a prescription than to talk," the physician explained. "I don't have enough time for an adequate dialogue."

This physician was most likely caught up in the vicious cycle of caring for too many patients without enough time to provide quality care.

At the same time, nurses are faced with long working hours and impossible patient assignments. Nurses have long struggled with health care inequities, and physicians have missed many opportunities to be supportive. Some physicians, feeling an alliance with nurses, have always been respectful. Others have been quick to devalue them.

Are physicians, CEOs, and other non-nurses finally ready put patients before their egos? Are physicians finally ready to acknowledge that they are not the only important professionals in health care? Don't we have enough health care challenges without unnecessary conflict?

Patients have lost opportunities to enjoy the benefits of trusting relationships with their caregivers. Healthful benefits inherent in these relationships give patients serenity and peace of mind. Illness is stressful enough without having to second-guess whether they can trust the intent of each physician, nurse, or manager.

Patients need consistency. Warm bonds with caregivers are healing in and of themselves. Consistency and relationships enable staff members do a better job. Caregivers lose effectiveness without a good understanding about a patient's personality, family, and personal values.

Medically complex procedures and lifesaving technologies do not replace the basic human need for love, caring, and compassion. Infants consistently become physically ill and even die if they receive only physical care without hearing the voice or feeling the touch of a parent or other caring person. Human beings continue to have these needs throughout their lives.

Regardless of one's heritage, people need spiritual as well as physical care. Recent data have suggested that our brains are wired for some form of spirituality. Various types of exercise, yoga, and even martial arts have been used for years to promote health. The parent of a child who won a contest to see who could stack the most Oreo cookies attributed his child's heightened sense of concentration to his tai chi training.

Studies about friendship describe its important health benefits for people of all ages. Some health care organizations have started promoting prayer. Meditation has been used for years to promote better physical and mental health.

Patients choose lifestyles and try to choose competent caregivers. Many times it is difficult for consumers to make those choices, because they face a myriad of data. When these data are public-relations hype, they are often slanted and distorted. Probably, the best way for consumers to choose caregivers is to develop trusting relationships with several health care professionals: physicians, nurses, or others. Ask them for recommendations. Use their suggestions and add their own thoughts and impressions. Schedule a "getting to know you" visit to discuss specific requests.

To make matters worse, patients seem to be adopting less healthy lifestyles, raising the rate of obesity-related diseases, substance abuse, and stress-related ailments. This makes it likely that our future will include even higher medical costs and greater demand for health services. Patients in countries with universal insurance endure long waits for elective procedures, or their wealthy patients use a parallel private-pay system.

Some organizations try to pass unreimbursed health care costs on to the uninsured. These patients—the working poor, the unemployed, young adults, or the self-employed—are the least able to bear this burden.

The ease of international travel has enabled global epidemics and medication-resistant organisms to become more dangerous. Pharmaceutical company policies and high prices make it difficult for the average person to discriminate between price gouging and legitimate costs of research.

World poverty, political conflict, and the need to share health resources beyond national borders complicate these issues even more.

As the baby boomers age, fewer nurses will be present to care for greater needs. This crunch will only get worse. Some reports indicate that we have enough nurses, but they have been driven out of health care by negative workplace environments.

Consumers have access to the Internet, which provides an abundance of medical information, yet the average consumer is unable to fully understand the data. They frequently aren't able to prioritize this information accurately or to use it to make intelligent decisions.

On the positive side, the Web is an important health-promotion tool. Consumers have used the Internet to assist their physicians with their care. Some families of patients with rare diseases have spent many hours researching information on the Web and have found lifesaving treatment protocols for their loved ones. Many physicians use Internet information for patient education. They refer specific sites as good sources for disease and medication information. The Web is a good source of health care research because there is an abundance of information available. In fact, one of the biggest problems to avoid is information overload.

MANAGED CARE: HAVING IT ALL—SAFETY, QUALITY, AND COST CONTROL

Consumers need the benefits that managed care (MC) organizations offer. More collaboration between medical professionals, consumers, and related health care industries would strengthen your health care system.

Managed care is the most promising way to solve our health care challenges—if it achieves its full potential. MC has the opportunity to capitalize on economies of scale with money, knowledge, and technology. Managed care organizations (MCOs) could provide the highest quality of care for the lowest possible cost.

Caring people, not policies and procedures, determine MC success. MC employees could be its greatest asset. Hiring a caring staff, giving them autonomy, and supporting them to provide quality services would allow MC to fulfill its promise. They could have it all—safety, quality, and cost control—and enjoy satisfied customers, profitability, and loyal employees.

MC is a matter of managing risk. Successful risk management starts with analyzing information. This chapter provides you with an overview of organizational, professional, and patient perspectives. It will suggest approaches to maximize MC's resources.

We have changed from a fee-for-service system to a capitated system whereby organizations assume risks for the total care needs for a specific number of people for a fixed amount of money. As with any service business, MC was expected to provide a service in return for payments by employers, individuals, and governmental agencies.

One of the problems that occurred with MC is that some MCOs tried to minimize the service they provided and maximize the payments they received. It's no different than a restaurant watering down its soup and losing its loyal customers, and it didn't take long for MCOs to lose consumer trust.

MC has become a nightmare for many people. A 2003 Gallup poll asked people what they thought were the most honest and respected professions. "Car salesman scored lowest in this year's poll, *followed by HMO managers*" [italics added] (AHA, 2003). Since nurses were rated the highest at 83% and MC managers were rated next to last, perhaps MC managers should ask nurses how to interact with customers and raise their score.

The MC bureaucracy and lack of accountability have become obstacles to health care reform. These obstacles will continue to exist until MCOs consider patient satisfaction as important as profitability.

Effective Managed Care

MC can provide invaluable services to consumers:

- Listening to patients
- Promoting preventative care

- Reducing expensive acute care
- Providing quality outcomes
- Individualizing care
- Focusing on high-touch as well as high-tech care
- Providing superior customer service
- Maintaining cost controls

Consider how MC broadens access to health care services:

1. Access to lifesaving care is available for patients who would otherwise find cutting-edge health care out of their reach. For example, a young couple starting out with a new home and new jobs give birth to a baby that needs care totaling $100,000. They would never have been able to provide this care without health insurance (managed care).

2. Access to skilled professionals who have the knowledge to guide patients through the illness process is available. For instance, an MC company assigns a case manager and health coach to a patient suffering from heart failure. Through teaching and medication management, this patient is able to reduce her emergency room visits by 50% percent over a 12-month period. She enjoys a higher level of health for the year, and her MC company was able to reduce its costs.

3. Access is available to preventative care that is not only cost-effective for treating disease, but also provides patients with a higher quality of life. Smokers have access to smoking cessation programs to improve their quality of life and reduce long-term medical costs.

4. Access to research enables patients to benefit from innovative treatments. A young child is able to receive a new treatment for cancer that saves his life. Research used by MC has made this possible.

5. Access is available to physicians who collaborate with skilled specialists, nurse practitioners, case managers, nurses and other professionals. They provide multidisciplinary care management. For example, a patient who was injured at work receives medical case-management services and advice from an orthopedic specialist. She recovers 25% faster and returns to work 2 weeks earlier.

When Managed Care Fails

1. An MCO denies preventive care and ends up paying much more for high acute care costs. An MCO denies weight-reduction treatment for an obese patient who is later hospitalized several times for cardiac conditions that could have been prevented by the weight loss.
2. An MCO takes so long to approve care that the patient's medical condition becomes worse. The resulting cost is twice what it would have been with timely approval. Example: A patient is denied hospital admission for a psychiatric illness. The illness escalates and the MC organization ends up paying more: high costs for an ER visit in addition to large hospitalization costs.
3. MC strays from its mission of providing quality service to patients and deny as many services as possible. Many states have passed laws that require maternity patients to have 48 hours of hospitalization instead of leaving after only 24 hours. Government intervention should never have been necessary.
4. An MCO denies alternative medicine measures that have been effective for certain patients. Suppose a patient finds relief from a spinal injury with acupuncture, but her MC company refuses coverage. She loses many workdays because other treatment has not been effective for her. Her acupuncture is less expensive than covered services, but it is still denied.
5. Unrealistic pressure on physicians to speed up their care reduces their ability to provide adequate treatment. Consider a physician who finds that he is unable to provide patients with even a minimum of quality care. He must see too many patients per hour. This caring physician retires early because his strong professional values about quality care remain unmet. Health care consumers have lost another well-qualified physician.
6. Inconsistent communication results in patient inconvenience. A patient needs care but has to spend many hours on the phone to ensure that his bills are paid. This interferes with his work hours and reduces his productivity.
7. Serving the bureaucracy instead of serving the patient: With little accountability to serve patients, the MC staff talk with patients who call, but keep transferring them from department to department without resolving any of their issues.

8. MCOs use a coercive approach to providers and prevent them from receiving fair reimbursement. Patients lose their local providers and have to drive long distances to other physicians and hospitals. If the contract that is offered to providers reimburses at such a low rate that the provider would lose money on each patient, the provider may pull out of the contract. Many patients would have to drive long distances to another provider.

Many non-nurses never realized the importance of nursing until so many departed from the health care industry. They never understood the real nature of nursing work until it remained undone. Now is a good time to become knowledgeable about nursing and learn how to effectively integrate nurses into health care.

PROMOTING COLLABORATION WITH OTHER PROFESSIONALS AND WITH PATIENTS

Tips for Clinical Nurses

> - Understand the CEO perspective
> - Build nurse/physician partnerships
> - Listen to what patients are saying
> - Read minutes of senior management's meetings if available
> - Look for ways to support positive managed-care initiatives

Tips for Managers

> - Support nurse/non-nurse collaboration
> - Communicate organizational vision to staff
> - Promote alignment of different management levels
> - Point out nursing's key role to organizational success
> - Assess employee attitudes

(continued)

Tips for Educators

- Include cost issues in your curriculum
- Update your own knowledge about non-nurse issues
- Dialogue with managed care professionals
- Be open-minded
- Encourage students to look at the big picture

CHAPTER 16

Becoming a Lifelong Learner: Accelerate Your Professional Development

Learners will inherit the earth while the learned will be wonderfully equipped to deal with a world that no longer exists.

—Eric Hoffer

Lifelong learning prepares nurses who are able to thrive in a constantly changing environment. Consider two universal truths: Knowledge is power and, When you stop learning you stop living.

Students are our future. New nurses will have an opportunity to determine the future of nursing by examining our system with fresh eyes. After training, they will be able to introduce new perspectives and needed reform.

Will our nursing education programs fulfill this promise? It is an awesome responsibility.

Students: Assess your nursing program by asking the following questions:

1. Does your nursing program encourage independent thinking?
2. Are you encouraged to use problem-solving strategies from other professions? For example, do you look at the methods

that engineers or marketing professionals use and compare them to health care approaches?

3. What communication and persuasive skills do you learn?
4. Are change management skills included in your curriculum?
5. When encouraged to maintain high standards, does your program give you specific ways about *how* you can accomplish this when you are assigned many more patients after graduation?
6. Are you encouraged to study group dynamics?
7. What experiences with other disciplines do you have? Do you know how other industries handle safety, customer satisfaction, and leadership? Have you talked with physical therapy, dieticians, and other health care professionals about the best ways to work together?
8. Are you encouraged to engage in self-reflection?
9. Is your critical thinking supported?
10. Are you learning leadership and management skills?

Health care needs nurse-education programs that prepare new graduates who are able to function well in their first jobs. Many health care facilities provide internships to assist new graduates in this transition. Internships have been a successful trend but operate better when new graduates come already well prepared.

Students need nursing instructors who are clinical role models and expert nurses themselves.

The best nursing programs form cooperative partnerships with a variety of clinical facilities: medical centers, nursing homes, adult day care centers, community health clinics, VNAs, and others. This arrangement provides many mutual advantages. The clinical facilities enrich their practice, and the nurse education programs profit from ready access to outstanding clinical experiences.

Clinical experience is extremely important because it forms the basis for making smart clinical decisions.

There are two ways to measure clinical experience. Suppose you meet a nurse with 10 years of experience. You will need to decide if that nurse has 1 year of experience repeated 10 times or actually has 10 years of experience.

Having 10 years of experience means that you have been willing to step out of your comfort zone whenever you have had an opportunity to learn. You will have used Smart Nursing strategies and viewed yourself as an asset to be developed. And you will have looked at your work from a long-term perspective.

This will enable you to exhibit excellent clinical judgment by using valuable clinical intuition. These skills are important to maintaining a solid patient-safety record because they enable you to make clinical decisions in a timely way.

Suppose you are a charge nurse and a patient seems to be developing some disturbing symptoms. The reality of patient care is that you don't have the luxury of waiting to obtain all the data you might like.

For example, you must make a decision before you have all the lab test results. You must decide whether to wait and assess further, whether to report the symptoms to the physician, or whether to operate in an emergency mode. Experienced clinical nurses are usually able to decide on the correct action to take.

If you are a new nurse, this is a good time to consult with an experienced nurse. And this is a reminder to learn from this experience and all of your own experiences so that you will eventually function as an experienced nurse. Remember that every nurse was a beginner when he or she first graduated.

The secret of fast learning is to volunteer to learn as much as possible. Volunteer to become IV certified; work to become certified in your specialty; plan to become ACLS certified if that designation is relevant to your work. Ask relevant questions. Volunteer to cross-train or develop a staff or patient education program. Take the initiative. Step outside your comfort zone. Develop a reputation of one who is consistently seeking professional growth.

You will reach various steps in the professional growth process. Reward yourself as you grow more competent, and use each new level to define your worth to your employer.

Not all employers understand the value of an experienced nurse and may need to be educated. One cause of the nursing shortage has been that many health care organizations have viewed nurses as being all the same. They think a nurse is a nurse is a nurse. They fail to understand that the presence of a clinically experienced nurse on the unit raises the number of correct clinical decisions. At the same time, experienced nurses assist novice nurses to develop sound professional judgment by supporting them with consistent coaching.

Experienced nurses sometimes resist this coaching role because it takes extra time, but accepting this important role is part of what makes experienced nurses valuable to their organization. Experienced nurses also will find that teaching novice nurses sharpens their own skills because teaching requires nurses to review the rationale of their practices.

Nurses should also educate their employers about the value of their coaching to novice nurses. Their coaching adds significant value to their organization. In other words, you add dollars and should be receiving some kind of reward for this work.

Many organizations use a system of clinical ladders to recognize higher levels of nursing excellence. With this approach, nurses with excellent clinical skills do not have to seek out management positions to earn more money and recognition. Most organizations recognize three levels of expertise, and the role of a clinical nurse III usually includes staff coaching, an expanded patient teaching role, and an expectation of solid critical thinking skills.

LEARN STRATEGIES FOR CHANGE

Look at your work environment to see how it could be better. Notice who is influential in your organization, and observe how they became effective. Make the following observations:

1. Do people introduce suggestions at staff meetings? Are they successful? What communication approach do they use?
2. Do they talk formally or informally with the nurse manager?
3. Do people put their requests in writing?
4. Do they seek out coworkers with similar perspectives and make suggestion as a group?
5. Have they presented suggestions at open meetings with the CEO? Were they effective?

Once you understand how successful change happens at your workplace, you will know what to do. Use your assessment and planning skills to become an effective change agent.

When you make a job change, start the observation process again because the politics at each facility are different. In each new job, spend at least 3 months observing the way that the new system works. Even positive cultures have personalities; they have certain ways to get things done. It is not a matter of good or bad; it's a matter of learning how your organization works. This observation method will enable you to identify quickly the strategies that successful people in that setting use.

THE VALUE OF INTELLECTUAL CAPITAL

Intellectual capital is one of your organization's most valuable assets, and it keeps on growing if managed well. We live in the information age.

You, as a new nurse, are part of your organization's capital. How you develop your skill sets will determine how much value you have to offer. If you use this currency well, your facility will become intellectually wealthy.

Intellectual capital includes work experience, specialized training, natural aptitudes of employees, non-nursing experience, and creativity.

Review the skills assessment in the appendix for a list of attributes important to personal and professional effectiveness. Broad skills enable nurses to become qualified clinicians, managers, and leaders. Skills especially important to influence others are public speaking, writing for publication, networking, and activity in professional associations. Articulate nurses are more likely to be heard.

The silence of nurses has been one of the main reasons for the nursing crisis. We have expected others to speak for us. No one has. We must find our voice and start speaking for ourselves.

Health care is a rapidly changing industry. Nurses who are avid students are able to retain their competency. You don't even have to enroll in an education program.

- Cultivate a sense of curiosity.
- Ask questions. When you meet other people, people from other industries as well, ask them how they approach their challenges. Then use an open mind to see if you can apply their techniques in health care.
- Go to your local library at least once a month.
- Check out a dozen books on a variety of subjects, and set aside a couple of hours to skim through them.
- Look for good ideas.
- Read a few chapters from your favorite books.

My experience has been that you will find something useful for health care in every single book. You will also be a good role model in lifelong learning for your peers and children.

Our world has changed, and so have the rules of the game. People have enjoyed long-term security in the past by working for the same organization. Now, the number of skills that you are able to exercise determines your job security, so your job security resides with you. Most important, since you have control of how many skills you learn, job security is an internal not external issue.

- Be proactive. Anticipate and embrace change rather than waiting to be forced. Rapid changes of census and acuity make cross training a fact of life. You have two choices: (a) Embrace cross training, and learn to do it well (positive); or (b) complain each time (negative).
- Brainstorm with your peers to identify emerging trends.
- Identify certain skills that have a particularly high return for your effort: Advanced Cardiac Life Support certification, IV certification, adult learning theory, CPR instructor certification and communication, leadership and management skills.
- Empower yourself with effective communication.
- Learn everything you can. When an opportunity to learn a new skill surfaces, volunteer right away. Accepting free training is always a smart decision. Become multiskilled as soon as possible.
- Expand your people skills so that you can function as an effective team leader. Listen to your team members with sensitivity.
- Notice superb team leaders, and observe how they interact with their team members.
- Read publications from both health care and non-health care industries. Broaden your perspective by exchanging information between disciples.
- Capitalize on diversity.

Consider the following example of successfully combining diverse viewpoints using education: An educator, who was asked to plan a program on innovation, decided to organize a panel that included four teams. Each team was composed of a natural innovator paired up with an influential long-term staff member. This exercise strengthened both people. The innovator became more influential and the long-term nurse more innovative. And the staff in the audience gained from the variety of participant perspectives.

Information from different industries and disciplines has common foundations. A breadth of knowledge enables you to apply basic ideas in a variety of different ways.

Use the following ideas to broaden your perspective:

- Ask "Why?" when you do something new.
- Then ask, "Does it make sense?"
- Think about ways to accomplish your work more simply while still achieving good results.
- Ask yourself if you have considered all of the possibilities. Talk with others to determine if they see situations differently.
- Cultivate an appreciation of novel thoughts and perspectives.
- Become a role model for personal and professional growth.
- Believe in yourself. Expect resistance from the status quo. Learn not to take negative feedback personally.
- Network (network everywhere).
- Cultivate an appreciation for other people.
- Develop expertise in small talk.
- Find good role models and learn from them.
- Limit your TV time and use that time for reading instead.
- Keep books in your car and read while you wait for appointments or when picking up your children.
- Read for 30 minutes every morning. That adds up to over 3 hours of reading every week. And it makes your day more focused.

As experienced patient interviewers, nurses already possess communication skills. They just need to reconfigure those communication skills to make them more versatile.

Health care is a labor-intensive industry, and money spent on human resources constitutes a large portion of a health care organization's budget. Staff development directors have an opportunity to leverage this large investment with strategic education programs.

Health care organizations need large numbers of competent nurses. They need nurses who are flexible, good at working in fast-paced environments, and competent in a wide variety of clinical areas. They need nurses who advocate for patient safety.

Imagine the difference if nurses were more assertive and articulate. What if nurses wrote articles, spoke to community groups, and influenced health care policies. Collectively, we have the knowledge, information, and compassion needed for health care reform.

PROMOTING FOR LIFELONG LEARNING

Tips for Clinical Nurses

- Think strategically
- Look for opportunities
- Keep your sense of humor
- Learn from your mistakes
- Cross train

Tips for Managers

- Support nurses' professional growth
- Recognize that nurses are high value human resources
- Consider nurses as assets
- Encourage knowledge sharing
- Support nurses who step out of their comfort zone

Tips for Educators

- Involve students in discussions about working with LPNs, LNAs, and others
- Build student self-confidence
- Discuss self-development challenges
- Promote flexibility
- Encourage students to take intelligent risks

CHAPTER 17

What Individual Nurses Can Do: How You Can Make a Difference

The best way to get what you want is to help the other side get what they want.

—Robert Shapiro

LOOK AT THE BIG PICTURE

Help management get what it wants so that nurses can get what they want. Conflict between nurse and management is needless, expensive and wasteful. Worst of all, it consumes time, talent, and money necessary for direct patient care.

Nurses and administrators share responsibility for this problem, but because this chapter focuses primarily on clinical nurses, it will point out how they can impact the nursing crisis by changing something about themselves.

Enlarge your thinking to include your CEO's viewpoint. You already know from communicating with patients that you must frame clinical suggestions around patient issues. Use the same principle when working with management—frame your requests around their important issues: safety, marketing, and financial success.

CEOs are responsible for your organization's survival. Issues that CEOs frequently consider to be important are (a) balancing the budget. Many payers reimburse less than the actual cost of care; (b)

183

expanding health care services into new markets; and (c) minimizing medical errors and risk.

Reframe Your Perspectives

Frame your comments from an articulate business point of view. Show how nursing adds value to your organization. Suppose you are a small community hospital with a wonderfully compassionate and competent nursing staff. An outstanding neurosurgeon from a nearby metropolitan area prefers to admit his patients to your hospital, mainly because of nursing excellence. Consider yourself as an important partner when talking with management. Comment on the value that nurses bring to the organization.

CEOs are beginning to realize that having enough good nurses is necessary for survival. This is new realization, because nurses have been undervalued in the past.

Point out that excellent patient care is an important factor that attracts patients to your facility. Patients tend to listen to their friends and neighbors when choosing health care facilities. Capitalize on that trend. Calculate your spin-off value as a premier marketer.

- Patients who are highly satisfied by their nursing care bring millions of dollars of revenue later on by recommending your facility to their friends and neighbors. And they are likely to return if they have further medical needs.
- Suppose a patient asks for a more homelike atmosphere in the hospital. This information is valuable input for management.
- Communicate a negative situation if it exists. Say, "The current short staffing is driving our patients away. Something needs to be done. We can't afford to keep losing patients. And, if the staffing remains low, we will be losing many nurses as well."

Look for Ways to Add Value to Your Organization

It is important to communicate this kind of information to your CEO and other managers. Focus on building bridges to a better future instead of only reiterating the past.

- Seek out councils, committees, or boards created to obtain nursing ideas.

- Initiate conversations with your VP of nursing to share mutual perspectives.
- Talk with committee members; examine written records and analyze their goals and actions.
- Inquire about joining an interdisciplinary group such as a customer satisfaction group, composed of many disciplines. Raise patient satisfaction by building relationships with a variety of professionals.
- Improve your communication skills so that you can effectively add substance to discussions. Learn negotiation skills so that you can be a player instead of a spectator.
- Focus on improving your critical thinking skills so that your suggestions become thoroughfares into the future instead of retreats into the past.
- Make a suggestion about new ways help your organization's success.

Initiate Partnerships with Management

Partnerships only work when management view nurses as valued professionals. Make the first move and build mutual respect.

I enrolled in my first business course, Accounting I, in 1983. My peers were surprised and wondered why a nurse working at a nonprofit health care facility would want to take an accounting course. They implied that a clinical nurse should focus only on clinical nursing issues. They thought that nurses should leave the business side of health care to management.

My perspective was different. I took accounting *because* my focus was on clinical issues. And my focus is *still* on clinical care. Improving patient care is one of my main reasons for writing this book.

Nurses cannot provide patients with adequate care unless they have enough resources—enough employees, supplies, and support staff. Part of our job is to communicate patient needs effectively to management. We must speak the language of business, articulate clinical needs, and understand our scarce resource environment.

Be Business Savvy

Nurses must be business savvy to obtain the necessary financial resources that drive quality care. Learning the language of business is a good first step.

When staffing is inadequate, point out (in business terms) that your facility can no longer afford the financial loss caused by short staffing. Consider the following suggestions:

- Short staffing causes nurses to find other jobs or leave the health care industry for good. Every time a nurse resigns, management loses more than $50,000.
- Short staffing increases the number of medical errors and raises your risk.
- Nurses are your greatest asset. Value them and treat them with respect.

Non-health-care organizations have succeeded by supporting the autonomy of frontline employees. Frontline employees are entrusted with the responsibility of satisfying the customers because they have the most customer contact. They become ambassadors for their companies. Companies who promote staff autonomy have been successful over time.

Be Accountable

Many nurses understandably are reluctant to accept greater accountability. They have been censured in the past for challenging the status quo, and they are reluctant to try again. But we must try again. Nurse autonomy is absolutely necessary if we hope to succeed in controlling health care costs and reducing medical errors. If management refuses to promote nurse autonomy, clinical nurses must educate management and be willing to demonstrate the benefits to their organization. Combine your clinical knowledge with solid persuasive skills to make sure that your recommendations to improve patient care are implemented.

Look to the future instead of repeating past practices. The nursing crisis may end up being just the right catalyst to transform health care problems into opportunities and actually improve health. Welcome difficult challenges. Nurses often engage in subtle avoidance behavior. They get sidetracked when confronted with problems. Instead of solving the main problem, they focus on the details first. Focusing on details is important, but first review the basic principles. Ask yourself, is this idea logical? Is it ethical? Will it improve patient care? Is it financially sound? Will the staff support it?

Be Willing to Change

Most progressive people step out of their comfort zones to achieve results. Change feels uncomfortable at first, but that discomfort is soon neutralized by the satisfaction of creating better practice. Use your knowledge and ability to create realistic solutions to health care challenges. Seek out control over your work. Learning new skills—communication, negotiation, and persuasion—will improve patient safety, increase nurse satisfaction, and raise productivity.

Nurses have lost power partly because we have neglected to become excellent communicators and negotiators. We have assumed that others would speak for us. No one has. Nurses are the ones who need to be articulate—learn to speak in public, write for publication, and negotiate effectively.

How? Join Toastmasters to learn public speaking. You will meet people who had been afraid to speak but have learned how to be well spoken. Join a writers group to learn how to write for publication. Read some books on negotiation. The same is true about writing for publication. A writing course or joining a writers group can enable you to have a second mode to express your views. What are your reasons for waiting? Too expensive? Most of these organizations are free. Some charge a nominal fee. You just need to act.

Some nurses say that they don't have time. This is understandable considering the large amount of overtime and other responsibilities. But nurses must take some initiative to stop the cycle of powerlessness and mandatory overtime. Learning new skills to become professionally articulate is the best way to address this vicious cycle.

Cross-train

Nurses have a huge effect on their organization's financial status due to the size of nursing budgets. Management has constraints from insurers, the government, and others. Nurses need to be flexible and willing to cross-train to help management achieve the best staff utilization. Remember, nurses become more successful when they help their whole organization succeed.

Work in different specialties to broaden your perspective. Network with other nurses and with people in other industries. Read widely. Avoid stagnating and getting in a rut. Be a lifelong learner.

Cross-training makes you a better nurse. Medical-surgical nurses who know psychiatry interact better with noncompliant or personality disordered patients. Nurses who understand home care plan better discharges. Ambulatory care nurses with managed care experience are better patient advocates.

Other cross training benefits are:

- Greater self-confidence
- Higher value to employers
- Better job prospects if you decide to change jobs

Know your limitations about being a safe clinician in new specialties. Be assertive in expressing your concerns if the proposed situation is potentially unsafe for patients or yourself.

Respect Others

Respect the LNAs (licensed nurse's aides). I present education programs to LNAs as well as nurses, and I sometimes hear that many nurses do not treat LNAs well. Are we treating other caregivers the same way that we have been treated? Be good role models. This means that

- We should treat LNAs with respect.
- Listen to their perspective. They spend much time with patients and have valuable information.
- Offer to assist LNAs when they need help. A good way to encourage nurse/LNA collaboration is to use nurse/LNA partnerships. Assign a group of patients to nurse/LNA partnerships. Expect joint accountability. It's time for nurses to value the contribution of all health care workers.
- Take time to teach LNAs how to improve their work, tactfully and with sensitivity.
- Use your sense of humor.

Use Tools Sensibly

We have many good tools but sometimes sabotage their effectiveness. When carried to the extreme, good tools become liabilities instead of assets. It's similar to patients who sometimes think if a little bit of medicine is good, a lot must be better. We know that this is not necessarily true. It is the same for nurses. Taking our tools to the extreme turns a positive tool into an obstacle.

Nursing care plans are a perfect example of frequent misuse of a good tool. When care plans were introduced in the 1980s, nurses on each shift either had to ask patients to describe their needs or discover them through an inconsistent reporting system. Many people wanted care plans to have a customized outline. Others wanted them to be more complete and initiated the era of standard care plans. We wrote care plans for every conceivable illness, laminated them, and inserted them into the Kardex. Because they were cumbersome and not individualized, nurses did not use them. We wasted a lot of time and money.

Some facilities use a hybrid version. It is a simplified guide that includes common nursing interventions for nurses to check off. Blank spaces are available to add interventions that were not included.

Multidisciplinary treatment planning is another good tool that is often misused. In the 1980s, the average psychiatric patient's length of stay was 2 to 3 weeks. Now it is often 2 to 3 days. However, the treatment-team planning process hasn't changed much. We should be able to write excellent plans in less time. One time, a nurse was the only one available to care for patients because the rest of the staff were at the treatment team meeting. Planning is important. But shouldn't our priority be actually giving the care? Effective nursing care plans and multidisciplinary treatment plans represent a significant opportunity to reduce expenses without decreasing quality.

Broaden Your Knowledge

Ideas are the new business capital. We should exchange good ideas among nursing, business, and education on a regular basis. Consider how the following scenarios illustrate the portability of skill sets between health care and other occupations.

A health care sales nurse decided to use SOAP notes to write sales reports (Subjective, Objective, Assessment, and Plan). As you may recall, SOAP notes are a clinical charting technique used by nurses and physicians. They are also versatile for many other kinds of reports. The sales manager considered SOAP note sales reports to be the best reports he had ever received. Compare the medical and sales examples using SOAP notes in Table 17.1.

History of SOAP Notes

According to Cameron (2002, p. 2), "SOAP notes are part of the problem-oriented medical records (POMR) approach most commonly used by physicians and other health care professionals. Developed by Weed (1964), SOAP notes are intended to improve the quality and continuity of client services by enhancing communication among health care professionals (Kettenbach, 1995) and by assisting them in better recalling the details of each client's case." (Ryback, 1974; Weed, 1971)

Critical paths are an example of how information can be transferred from another industry to health care. Critical paths are often considered by health care professionals as a new idea of the 1990s. However, critical paths were adapted for use in health care only after they had been used in other industries for many years. Critical paths were used in engineering for more than 20 years before they were used in health care.

TABLE 17.1   SOAP Notes

	Medical Example	Sales Example
S	Patient says, "My stress at work has increased."	Customer says, "We aren't getting our shipments on time."
O	Patient's blood pressure is 150/90.	Customer order sheets are correct and faxed on time.
A	Difficulty coping with company downsizing.	Orders received on Mondays are delayed.
P	Try scheduled rest breaks and exercise for relaxation.	Try rescheduling order-takers on Mondays to avoid shipment delays.

Why don't we transfer information between disciplines more often? Why don't nurses network with people from other industries? If nurses would ask other professionals how they solve their problems, nurses could adapt some of those ideas to health care.

Are you willing to analyze your attitude and behavior? Will you make any necessary changes? Making changes may be easier than you think. And the rewards are great, because it is a well-known fact that people who continue to grow and evolve through their whole lives experience more happiness.

Tracing the History of Critical Paths

According to Bryant (1995):

> Peg A. Hofman, RN, TQM Coordinator at Mount Clemons General Hospital, traced the beginning of the critical path method to the mid-1950s. . . . At that time annual maintenance projects in the oil and chemical refinery industry were plotted on layouts from start to finish in a timeline that gave a "big picture" visualization.
>
> In industry, it has proven to be a valuable tool for charting projects that require the coordination of hundreds of separate contractors; it is commonly used in engineering, construction, and computer work. The earliest use of CPM reported in health care literature was in the mid-1980s by Zander, who adopted the CPM concept to review the delivery of patient care at the New England Medical Center, in Boston. The technique has been adapted to coordinate projects in both product and service organizations. (p. 3)

In 1991, Grudich reported a major improvement in operating room efficiency by applying CPM at St. Cloud Hospital in Minnesota. In 1992, the term *critical path* first appeared as a major heading in the index for *Nursing and Allied Literature.*

My question is this: Why did it take more than 30 years for health care to adopt critical paths? I think the answer is that health care organizations failed to understand how much they could learn from others.

If health care leaders and clinical workers had networked with those in engineering and the military and with others using critical paths, health care agencies could have enjoyed the benefits of this very useful technique much sooner.

PROMOTING INDIVIDUAL NURSING ACTION

Tips for Clinical Nurses

- Look at the big picture
- Be willing to step out of your comfort zone
- Work toward positive change with your peers
- Evaluate the effectiveness of your interventions
- Support your own personal growth

Tips for Managers

- Encourage clinical nurses to get involved in the change process
- Value nurse contributions
- Highlight staff nurse change efforts on their evaluations
- Facilitate group efforts for improvements
- Maximize staff efforts to improve productivity

Tips for Educators

- Chart a postgraduate self-development plan
- Include change management in your curriculum
- Be forward thinking
- Support community-building skills
- Coordinate future needs in your program

APPENDIX

Skill Assessment

Learnable/ Transferable Skills	*Styles to Develop*
Public Speaking	Energetic
Networking	Attention to detail
CPR Instructor	Gets along well with
Venipuncture skills	people
Clinical skills (cross-	Determined
training)	Works well under
Certifications	pressure
Leadership skills	Sensitive
Management skills	Intuitive
Conducts research	Persistent
Storytelling	Dynamic
Education theory	Dependable
Writing	Flexible
Knowledge of legal	Creative/innovative
system	Problem-solving
Computer competence	_____
Efficient reading with	_____
comprehension	_____
Acting	
Artistic abilities	Mark the skills that you al-
Musical talent	ready have with an X.
Mediation/diplomacy	Then circle three skills
Graduate degree	that you would like to de-
Financial expertise	velop. ADD other relevant
Strategic planning	skills and/or qualities in
_____	the blank spaces to cus-
_____	tomize the list.
_____	

CHAPTER 18

Through the Process
of Change Emerges the Decade
of the Nurse

Nancy M. Valentine

Despite the clamor regarding the many contemporary challenges to the nursing profession such as the nurse shortage, stressful working conditions, and difficulties attracting young, bright people to the field, one of the paradoxes is that many are beginning to recognize that this may be the *Decade of the Nurse*. How can that be possible with shrinking enrollments, a shortage that is expected to rise to 500,000 fewer personnel than needed by 2012, and nurses bargaining for legislated staffing patterns?

The answer may lie in how these facts are translated to the public and how the profession is marketed to aspiring nurses and to those in practice. All of the trends mentioned are factually correct, but how might this information be received if packaged differently where there was more emphasis on the positive?

For instance, there is a real nurse shortage, but one of the reasons, often not discussed, is that there is a vibrant increase in demand for nursing talent. Having lived through the 1980s and 1990s where nurse substitution, using so-called patient-centered approaches largely failed, there is greater recognition among health care leaders and the public that the skills and talents of a nurse simply cannot be interchanged with well-meaning personnel trained on the job. As regulatory agencies have more actively addressed the patient safety

194

issues in health care, there is clearer recognition that nurses are on the front lines and play the most critical of all roles in establishing and maintaining patient safety. But do we receive that recognition in all of the patient safety initiatives that have been put forward since the Institute of Medicine's report on patient safety?

The fact is jobs have expanded, particularly in nontraditional settings. Payers, pharmaceutical companies, and biotechnical companies have involved more nurses in their customer-focused products, ethical conduct of clinical trials, and sales initiatives targeted to professionals in delivery networks. As a result, nurses have migrated into important business environments in large numbers. The image of the nurses has not expanded accordingly, as we seem locked into traditional delivery settings at the bedside, whereas nursing roles have quietly expanded to every aspect of health care.

Yes, there are demographic aspects of an aging nurse workforce that are contributing significantly to the current shortage. Yet, if we could more effectively communicate the immense range of opportunities and forums where nurses make a difference every day, we would have a better chance of marketing our chosen profession. For many young people who have a wide range of career options and are often not familiar with the details of the field, the narrow focus on shortages and related work environment issues is heard by the listener as a negative endorsement. Such messages translate to a profession that is thought to be unappealing, hence contributing to shrinking growth of the profession.

What can we do? Many innovative ideas are needed. For example, marketing nursing to young people will need to be reinvented. We must revamp the image of solely appealing to those who can "tolerate the sight of blood." An image of nursing that more accurately describes the range of possibilities would increase demand for more nurse programs, not less. We could expand the pool of potential applicants by positioning the nursing major as mainstream, not for those simply willing to carry bedpans.

With an understanding that nursing is very broad, rather than narrowly defined, the nursing major could be repositioned as a fundamental course of study, as preparatory for life, and as a respectable profession and a basic pathway to advanced study in other fields. If marketed as an option with potentially more appeal than a liberal arts degree, for example, we would have many more colleges and universities screening potential students for the nursing major and mainstreaming students into this course of study. Increasing the number of applicants through such channels would increase the number of the best-qualified candidates for the profession.

We need to market career positives. Nursing has many advantages that other fields do not offer, such as flexible hours, improved salary options, and meaningful work that involves both scientific and humanitarian aspects. Nursing has one of the highest participation rates of any profession, meaning that those who are trained continue to work for many years after completing their initial course of study. One of the reasons for this is that there are so many opportunities for nurses to practice and remain in the workforce, long after retirement eligibility. Many continue employment because they enjoy their work and find opportunities throughout their communities to utilize their highly transferable skills.

Highlighted by the advent of the advanced practice nurse, there is growing awareness among the public the contributions of nurses. Public opinion polls consistently rate nursing the highest scores in public trust. This is a great honor as well as a responsibility. Information such as this needs to be shared more broadly.

We have to find better ways of describing and promoting the opportunities that already exist and create a vision and speak passionately as to how nurses are major players in redefining health care in the United States. This is less a vision of the future and more a reality of what actually exists today. We need to find our inspiring contemporary leaders in the field and give them more exposure to tell their stories.

As a personal example, when I was a young teen, I volunteered at a local hospital and knew from that experience that nursing was the career for me. Early on I aspired to be a good hospital nurse and focused my energies on acquiring the coveted technical skills. As I embarked on my career path, I touched patients and families in hospitals, in their homes, and in their communities. Later, I taught students, created a safe environment for research subjects, and learned about policy and politics and how these influence nursing practice. Having acquired additional knowledge in management, public health, and health care financing, I eventually found how transferable the nursing process and other skills were to complex environments in health care, government, and business.

Could I have known these possibilities when I started out? Very unlikely. Stories of nurse trailblazers were, in my early experience, limited to Florence Nightingale and nurses on horseback in the back woods of Kentucky. If we could find our collective voices to sing the praises of our life's work, we could communicate our mission more vividly to a public eager to listen. The opportunity is now and we must take advantage of it.

Epilogue

It is time to create health care environments that allow nurses to **work smart** and to remove the obstacles that prevent nurses from using their **full professional capacities. We owe it to our patients, and we owe it to ourselves.**

Remember the adage "Give a man a fish, and you feed him for a day. Teach him how to fish, and you feed him for a lifetime."

Smart Nursing gives you a system of proven practices that encourages you to add your own input. It promotes cost-effective solutions; in fact, there are more than 500 no-cost suggestions available for your use.

We hope that Smart Nursing brings people together. All health care workers are important—managers of all levels and nurses, whatever their preparation. Physicians, trustees, and other non-nurses; professionals in other disciplines such as OT, PT, pharmacy, and dietary; and paraprofessionals should have input.

We need everyone's input. Learn to work together. Get in the habit of viewing challenges as opportunities. Become a lifelong learner.

Patients deserve our best efforts. When we provide it we will once again be able to look each other in the eye and say, "Congratulations on a job well done."

In conclusion: Take action.

Recommended Reading

Benner, P. (1984). *From novice to expert, excellence and power in clinical nursing practice*. Addison-Wesley: New York: Reading, MA.

Brown, M. T. (1990). *Working Ethics: Strategies for decision making and organizations responsibility*. San Francisco: Jossey-Bass.

Collins, J. (2001). *Good to great*. New York: Harper Collins.

Connors, R. (1994). *The OZ principle*. Paramus, NJ: Prentice Hall.

Dawson, R. (1993). *The confident decision maker*. New York: William Morrow.

Dawson, R. (1995). *Roger Dawson's secrets of power negotiation*. The Career Press.

Dolan, J. P. (1992). *Negotiate like the pros*. New York: Berkley Publishing Group.

Fisher, R. (1981). *Getting to yes*. New York: Penguin Books.

Goleman, D. (2002). *Primal leadership*. Boston: Harvard Business School Press.

Hendricks, G. (1996). *The corporate mystic*. New York: Bantam Books.

Katzenbach, J. (1993). *The wisdom of teams*. New York: Harper Collins.

Koch, R. *The 80/20 principle*. (1998). The secret of achieving more with less. New York: Doubleday.

Lancaster, L. (2002). *When generations collide*. New York: Harper Business.

Landau, S., et al. (2001). *From conflict to creativity*. San Francisco: Jossey-Bass.

Lightfoot-Lawrence, S. (1999). *Respect*. Reading, MA: Perseus Books.

Mitchell, W. (1997). *It's not what happens to you; it's what you do about it*. Denver, CO: Phoenix Press.

Morrissey, J. (2002). Following nurses' orders. *Modern Healthcare, 32*(34), 36.

Needleman, J., Buerhaus, P., Mattke, S., Stewart, M., Zelevinsky, K. (2002). Nurse staffing levels and the quality of care in hospitals. *New England Journal of Medicine, 346,* 1715–1720.

Nursing Executive Center. (2000). *Reversing the flight of talent: Nursing retention in an era of gathering shortage*. Washington, DC: The Advisory Board Company.

Peck, M. S. (1978). *The road less traveled. A new psychology of love, traditional values and spiritual growth*. New York: Simon & Schuster.

Reinhold, B. (1996). *Toxic work*. New York: Penguin.

Roane, S. (1997). *What do I say next?* New York: Warner Books.

Rosen, E. (2000). *The anatomy of buzz*. New York: Random House.

Senge, P. (1990). *The fifth discipline: The art and practice of the learning organization*. New York: Doubleday.

Shapiro, R. M. (1998). *The power of nice.* New York: John Wiley & Sons.

Tieman, J. (2002). Study: Docs contribute to the nursing shortage. *Modern Healthcare, 32*(24).

Upenieks, V. (2003). What constitutes effective leadership? *J Nurs Adm, 33,* 456–467.

Wilson, E. O. (1998). *Consilience, The unity of knowledge.* New York: Knopf.

Work Environment for Nurses and Patient Safety. Website: www.nih.gov.

Zukav, G. (1989). *The seat of the soul.* New York: Fireside Books.

References

Aiken, L. H., Clarke, S. P., Silber, J. H., & Sloane, D. (2003, October). Hospital nurse staffing, education, and patient mortality. *LDI Issue Brief, 9*(2), 2–3.

American Health Care Association (AHCA). Website: www.ahca.org. Retrieved January 5, 2004.

American Hospital Association (AHA) (2003). News. December 15, 2003. p. 16.

American Nurses' Association (ANA). Website: www.nursingworld.org. Retrieved 2003.

Australian. www.theaustralian.news.com.au.

Brown, M. (1990). *Working ethics: Strategies for decision making and organizations' responsibility.* San Francisco: Jossey-Bass.

Bryant, M. R. (1995). Critical pathways: What they are and what they are not. *Tar Heel Nurse, 57*(5), 18.

Buresh, B., & Gordon, S. (2000). *From silence to voice.* Ottawa: Canadian Nurses Association.

Cameron, S. (2002). Learning to write case notes using SOAP format. *Journal of Counseling & Development, 80*(3), 2.

Dawson, R. (1993). *The confident decision maker.* New York: William Morrow.

Gallup. Website: http://www.gallup.com. Retrieved February 15, 2004.

Goleman, D. (2002). *Primal leadership.* Boston: Harvard Business School Press.

Institute of Medicine (IOM). Keeping patients safe: Transforming the work environment of nurses. Website: www.ion.edu. Retrieved February 15, 2004.

Jessee, W. (2003). It's time for a change. *Modern Healthcare, 33*(41), 26.

Johannes, L. (2002, May 30). Serious health risks posed by lack of nurses. *The Wall Street Journal,* pp. D1, D3.

Joint Commission on Accreditation of Health Care Organizations (JCAHO). Patient safety: Instilling hospitals with a culture of continuous improvement. Website: www.jcaho.org. Retrieved December 21, 2004.

Kaye, B. (2003, April). From assets to investors. *T & D, 57*(4).

Koch, R. (1998). *The 80/20 principle: The secret of achieving more with less.* New York: Doubleday.

Lancaster, L. (2002). *When generations collide.* New York: Harper Business.

Landau, S., et al. (2001). *From conflict to creativity.* San Francisco: Jossey-Bass.

Mitchell, W. (1997). *It's not what happens to you: It's what you do about it.* Denver, CO: Phoenix Press.

Morrissey, J. (2002). Following nurses' orders. *Modern Healthcare, 32*(34), 36.

National Institute of Health (NIH). Website: www.nih.gov. Retrieved February 15, 2004.

Needleman, J., Buerhaus, P., Mattke, S., Stewart, M., Zelevinsky, K. (2002). Nurse staffing levels and the quality of care in hospitals. *New England Journal of Medicine, 346*, 1715–1720.

New York Times. Editorial (2002). "Dying for lack of nurses," *10*(25).

Nurses top Gallup's Ethical Standards List (2003). AHA News (December 15), p. 16.

Nursing Executive Center. (2000). *Reversing the flight of talent. Nursing retention in an era of gathering shortage.* Washington, DC: The Advisory Board Company.

O'Sullivan, A. (2001, June). Statement for the Committee on Governmental Affairs Subcommittee on Oversight of Government Management, Restructuring, and the District of Columbia on Addressing Direct Care Staffing Shortages. Presented for the American Nurses Association from the Nursing World Website: http://nursingworld.org/gova/federal/legis/testimon/2001/GOVAREF. HTM. Retrieved July 28, 2004.

Peck, M. S. (1978). *The Road Less Traveled: A New Psychology of Love, Traditional Values, and Spiritual Growth.* New York: Simon & Schuster.

Reinhold, B. B. (1996). *Toxic work.* New York: Penguin.

Roane, S. (1997). *What do I say next?* New York: Warner Books.

Rosen, E. (2000). *The anatomy of buzz.* New York: Random House.

Senge, P. (1990). *The fifth discipline: The art and practice of the learning organization.* New York: Doubleday.

Stanley, T. (2000). *The millionaire mind.* Kansas City: Andrews McMeel Publishing.

Tieman, J. (2002). Study: Docs contribute to the nursing shortage. *Modern Healthcare, 32*(24), 26.

Tucker, A. L., Edmonson, A. C., & Spear, S. (2002). When problem solving prevents organizational learning. *Journal of Organizational Change Management, 15*(2), 135.

Upenieks, V. (2003). What constitutes effective leadership? *Journal of Nursing Administration, 33*, 456–467.

Weiss, A. (2000). Leadership for the new millennium. Website: www.summit consulting.com. Retrieved on January 2002.

Welch, J. (2001). *Jack: Straight from the gut.* New York: Warner Books.

Zukav, G. (1989). *The seat of the soul.* New York: Fireside Books.

Index